If found, please return to:

Copyright © 2020 Soulpress

No part of this book may be reproduced or used in any
manner without written permision of the copyright owner
except for the use of quotations in a book review.

Dear self,

Before embarking on this journey of self awareness and self love, I'd like to tell you a few things:

First of all, thank you for deciding to love and take care of yourself. Well done! I am so proud of you, especially knowing your super busy schedule.

Secondly, please don't forget that good things take time. It's not like you plant a seed at night and wake up the next day to a tree. Sure, sometimes things won't go the way you want them to, and sometimes you'll may feel like giving up, but even when that happens, just keep going. You'll thank me later.

Last but not least, I'd like to remind you that you are beautiful the way you are. Skinny. Curvy. Chubby. It doesn't matter. It's not like you're not liking or accepting yourself. No, that's not it. It's just that, now, you're aspiring to become a healthier, fitter, and stronger version of yourself. And I can't wait to see it.

With love,

This is me, at my starting point

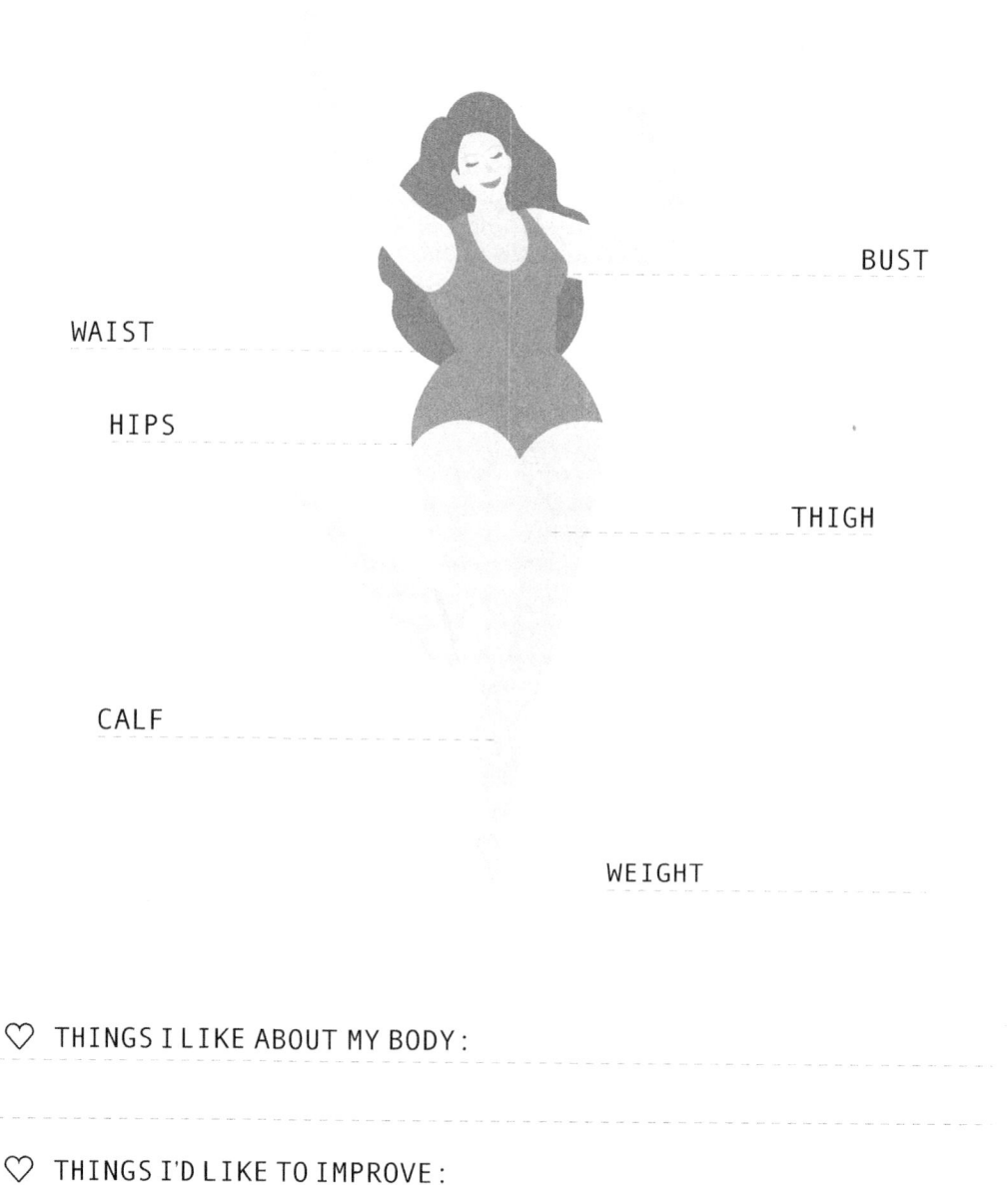

BUST

WAIST

HIPS

THIGH

CALF

WEIGHT

♡ THINGS I LIKE ABOUT MY BODY:

♡ THINGS I'D LIKE TO IMPROVE:

Goals for my mind, body & soul

GOALS:

MEASUREMENTS

BUST

WAIST

HIPS

THIGH

CALF

WEIGHT

GOOD HABITS TO BUILD:

BAD HABITS TO CUT:

MOTIVATION - WHAT KEEPS ME GOING:

Progress tracker

―――――― KEEP TRACK OF YOUR HABITS ――――――

WEEK 1	♡1 ♡2 ♡3 ♡4 ♡5 ♡6 ♡7
WEEK 2	♡8 ♡9 ♡10 ♡11 ♡12 ♡13 ♡14
WEEK 3	♡15 ♡16 ♡17 ♡18 ♡19 ♡20 ♡21
WEEK 4	♡22 ♡23 ♡24 ♡25 ♡26 ♡27 ♡28
WEEK 5	♡29 ♡30 ♡31 ♡32 ♡33 ♡34 ♡35
WEEK 6	♡36 ♡37 ♡38 ♡39 ♡40 ♡41 ♡42
WEEK 7	♡43 ♡44 ♡45 ♡46 ♡47 ♡48 ♡49
WEEK 8	♡50 ♡51 ♡52 ♡53 ♡54 ♡55 ♡56
WEEK 9	♡57 ♡58 ♡59 ♡60 ♡61 ♡62 ♡63
WEEK 10	♡64 ♡65 ♡66 ♡67 ♡68 ♡69 ♡70
WEEK 11	♡71 ♡72 ♡73 ♡74 ♡75 ♡76 ♡77
WEEK 12	♡78 ♡79 ♡80 ♡81 ♡82 ♡83 ♡84
WEEK 13	♡85 ♡86 ♡87 ♡88 ♡89 ♡90

―――――― COLOR KEY ――――――

♡ COMPLETE   ♡ INCOMPLETE   ♡ SKIPPED

DAY 1

One day or day one?

BREAKFAST

WEIGHT

LUNCH

WATER

○ ○ ○ ○
○ ○ ○ ○

DINNER

SNACKS

EXERCISE

SLEEP TIME

TODAY I AM GRATEFUL FOR:

MOOD TODAY

DAY 2

BREAKFAST

WEIGHT

LUNCH

WATER

○ ○ ○ ○
○ ○ ○ ○

DINNER

SNACKS

EXERCISE

SLEEP TIME

THIS SONG MAKES ME HAPPY :

MOOD TODAY

DAY 3

BREAKFAST

WEIGHT

LUNCH

WATER

○ ○ ○ ○
○ ○ ○ ○

DINNER

SNACKS

EXERCISE

SLEEP TIME

POSITIVE AFFIRMATIONS:

MOOD TODAY

DAY 4

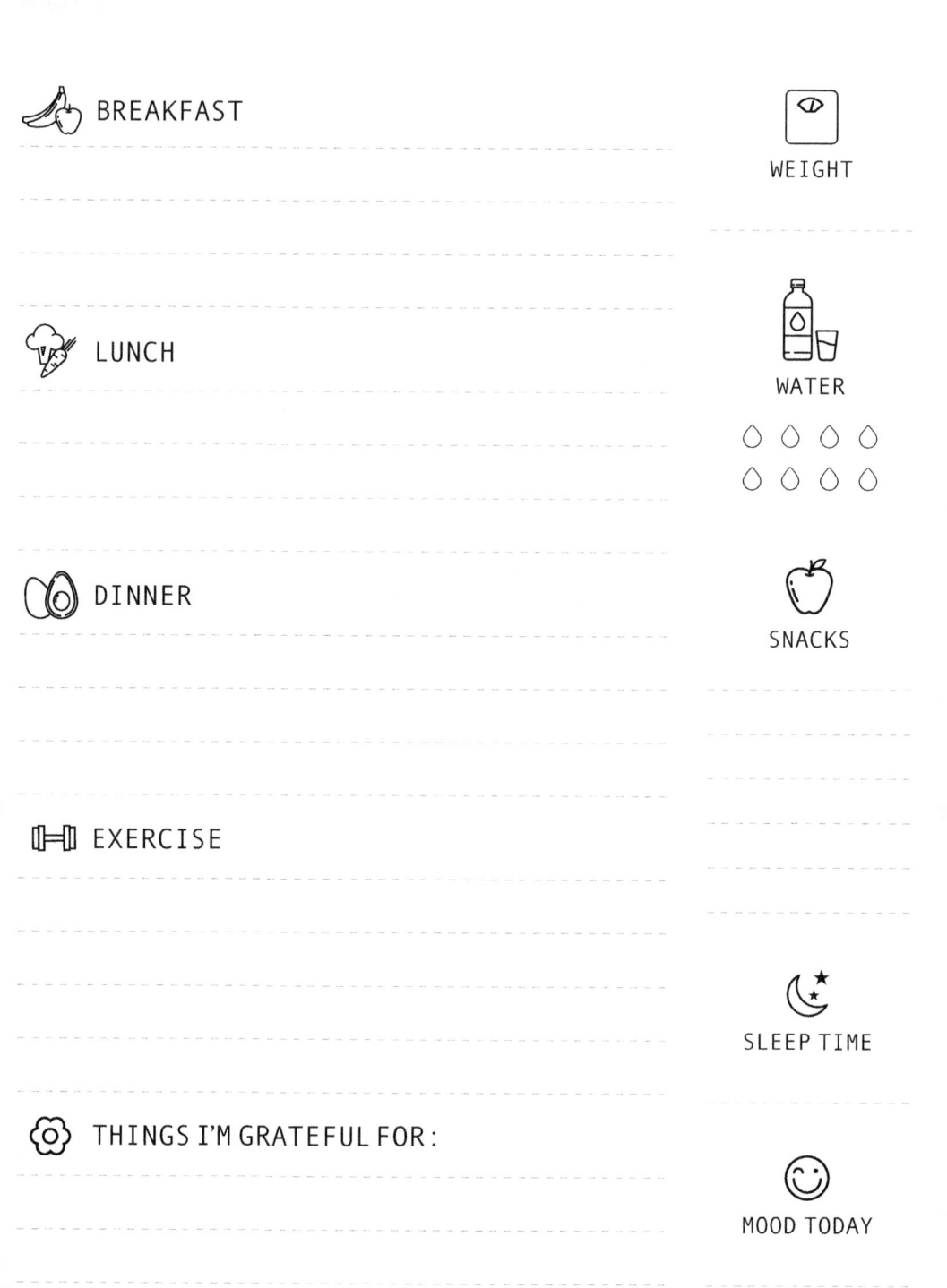

BREAKFAST

LUNCH

DINNER

EXERCISE

THINGS I'M GRATEFUL FOR:

WEIGHT

WATER

○ ○ ○ ○
○ ○ ○ ○

SNACKS

SLEEP TIME

MOOD TODAY

DAY 5

Wake up beauty. It's time to beast.

BREAKFAST

LUNCH

DINNER

EXERCISE

THIS PERSON INSPIRES ME:

WEIGHT

WATER

○ ○ ○ ○
○ ○ ○ ○

SNACKS

SLEEP TIME

MOOD TODAY

DAY 6

BREAKFAST

WEIGHT

LUNCH

WATER

○ ○ ○ ○
○ ○ ○ ○

DINNER

SNACKS

EXERCISE

SLEEP TIME

QUOTE OF THE DAY:

MOOD TODAY

DAY 7

BREAKFAST

WEIGHT

LUNCH

WATER

○ ○ ○ ○
○ ○ ○ ○

DINNER

SNACKS

EXERCISE

SLEEP TIME

TODAY'S MANTRA:

MOOD TODAY

DAY 8

BREAKFAST

WEIGHT

LUNCH

WATER

○ ○ ○ ○
○ ○ ○ ○

DINNER

SNACKS

EXERCISE

SLEEP TIME

MY HOPES FOR TOMORROW:

MOOD TODAY

DAY 9

Think it. Want it. Get it.

BREAKFAST

WEIGHT

LUNCH

WATER

○ ○ ○ ○
○ ○ ○ ○

DINNER

SNACKS

EXERCISE

SLEEP TIME

A BOOK THAT INSPIRES ME:

MOOD TODAY

DAY 10

BREAKFAST

WEIGHT

LUNCH

WATER

○ ○ ○ ○
○ ○ ○ ○

DINNER

SNACKS

EXERCISE

SLEEP TIME

ONE ACT OF KINDNESS:

MOOD TODAY

DAY 11

BREAKFAST

WEIGHT

LUNCH

WATER

○ ○ ○ ○
○ ○ ○ ○

DINNER

SNACKS

EXERCISE

SLEEP TIME

TODAY'S MANTRA:

MOOD TODAY

DAY 12

BREAKFAST

LUNCH

DINNER

EXERCISE

MY STRENGTHS :

WEIGHT

WATER

○ ○ ○ ○
○ ○ ○ ○

SNACKS

SLEEP TIME

MOOD TODAY

DAY 13

Prove them wrong.

BREAKFAST

WEIGHT

LUNCH

WATER

○ ○ ○ ○
○ ○ ○ ○

DINNER

SNACKS

EXERCISE

SLEEP TIME

BEST THING THAT HAPPENED TO ME :

MOOD TODAY

DAY 14

BREAKFAST

WEIGHT

LUNCH

WATER

○ ○ ○ ○
○ ○ ○ ○

DINNER

SNACKS

EXERCISE

SLEEP TIME

A PLACE THAT I LOVE:

MOOD TODAY

DAY 15

BREAKFAST

LUNCH

DINNER

EXERCISE

QUOTE OF THE DAY:

WEIGHT

WATER

SNACKS

SLEEP TIME

MOOD TODAY

DAY 16

BREAKFAST

WEIGHT

LUNCH

WATER

DINNER

SNACKS

EXERCISE

SLEEP TIME

A GOOD THING I DID TODAY:

MOOD TODAY

DAY 17

One step at a time.

🍌 BREAKFAST

🥦 LUNCH

🥑 DINNER

🏋 EXERCISE

⚙ TODAY'S GOALS:

⚖ WEIGHT

💧 WATER
○ ○ ○ ○
○ ○ ○ ○

🍎 SNACKS

🌙 SLEEP TIME

☺ MOOD TODAY

DAY 18

BREAKFAST

LUNCH

DINNER

EXERCISE

SIMPLE PLEASURES I ENJOY:

WEIGHT

WATER

SNACKS

SLEEP TIME

MOOD TODAY

DAY 19

BREAKFAST

LUNCH

DINNER

EXERCISE

POSITIVE AFFIRMATIONS:

WEIGHT

WATER

○ ○ ○ ○
○ ○ ○ ○

SNACKS

SLEEP TIME

MOOD TODAY

DAY 20

BREAKFAST

WEIGHT

LUNCH

WATER

DINNER

SNACKS

EXERCISE

SLEEP TIME

THINGS I LIKE ABOUT MY BODY:

MOOD TODAY

DAY 21

Think happy. Stay happy.

BREAKFAST

LUNCH

DINNER

EXERCISE

THINGS TO DO BETTER:

WEIGHT

WATER

○ ○ ○ ○
○ ○ ○ ○

SNACKS

SLEEP TIME

MOOD TODAY

DAY 22

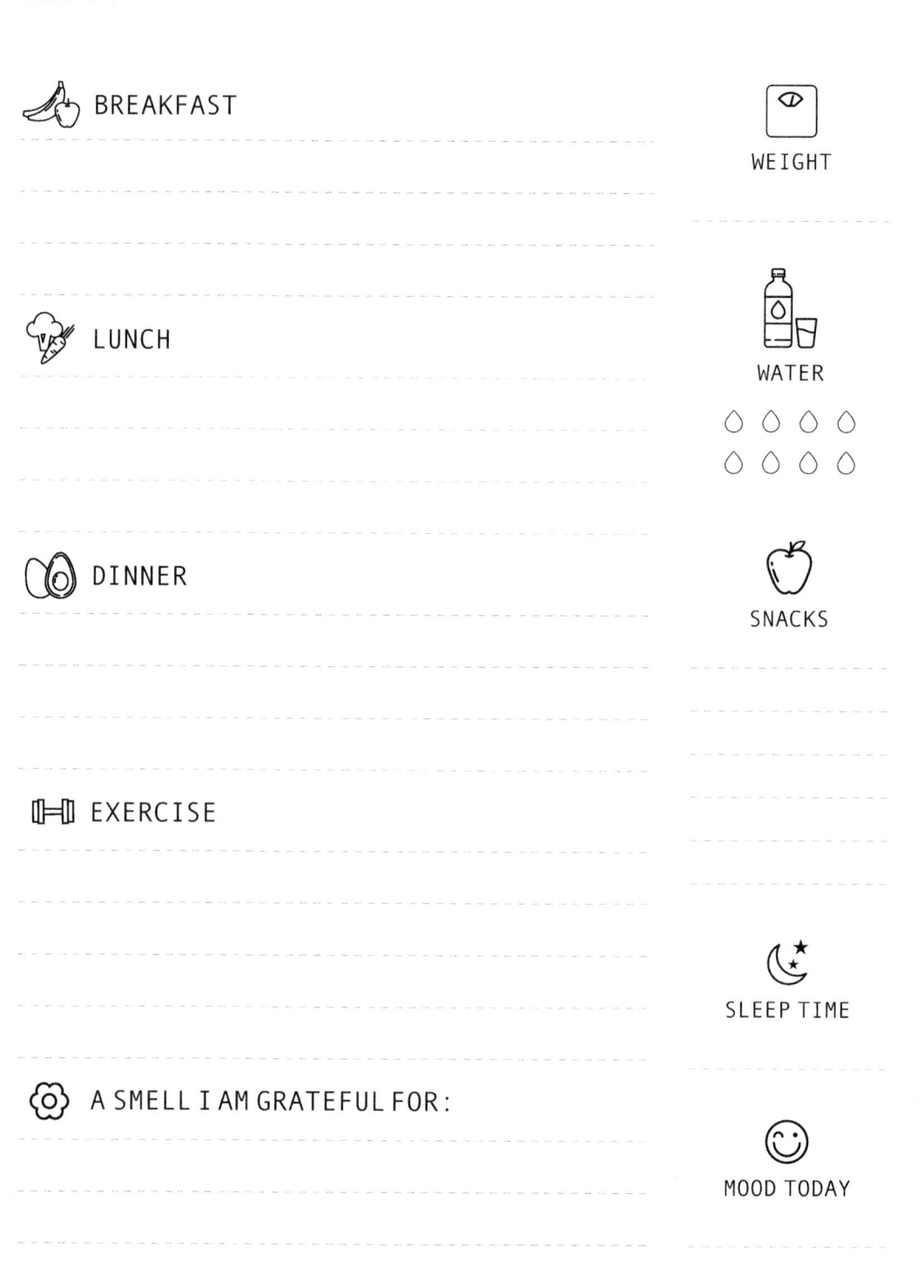

BREAKFAST

WEIGHT

LUNCH

WATER

○ ○ ○ ○
○ ○ ○ ○

DINNER

SNACKS

EXERCISE

SLEEP TIME

A SMELL I AM GRATEFUL FOR:

MOOD TODAY

DAY 23

BREAKFAST

LUNCH

DINNER

EXERCISE

REFLECTIONS ON THE DAY:

WEIGHT

WATER

SNACKS

SLEEP TIME

MOOD TODAY

DAY 24

BREAKFAST

WEIGHT

LUNCH

WATER

○ ○ ○ ○
○ ○ ○ ○

DINNER

SNACKS

EXERCISE

SLEEP TIME

TODAY I AM GRATEFUL FOR:

MOOD TODAY

DAY 25

You are your only limit.

🍌 BREAKFAST

🥦 LUNCH

🥑 DINNER

🏋 EXERCISE

🌸 THINGS I LIKE ABOUT MYSELF:

WEIGHT

WATER

○ ○ ○ ○
○ ○ ○ ○

SNACKS

SLEEP TIME

MOOD TODAY

DAY 26

BREAKFAST

WEIGHT

LUNCH

WATER

○ ○ ○ ○
○ ○ ○ ○

DINNER

SNACKS

EXERCISE

SLEEP TIME

GOOD THINGS ABOUT TODAY:

MOOD TODAY

DAY 27

BREAKFAST

LUNCH

DINNER

EXERCISE

QUOTE OF THE DAY:

WEIGHT

WATER
○ ○ ○ ○
○ ○ ○ ○

SNACKS

SLEEP TIME

MOOD TODAY

DAY 28

BREAKFAST

WEIGHT

LUNCH

WATER

DINNER

SNACKS

EXERCISE

SLEEP TIME

FOOD I AM MOST GRATEFUL FOR:

MOOD TODAY

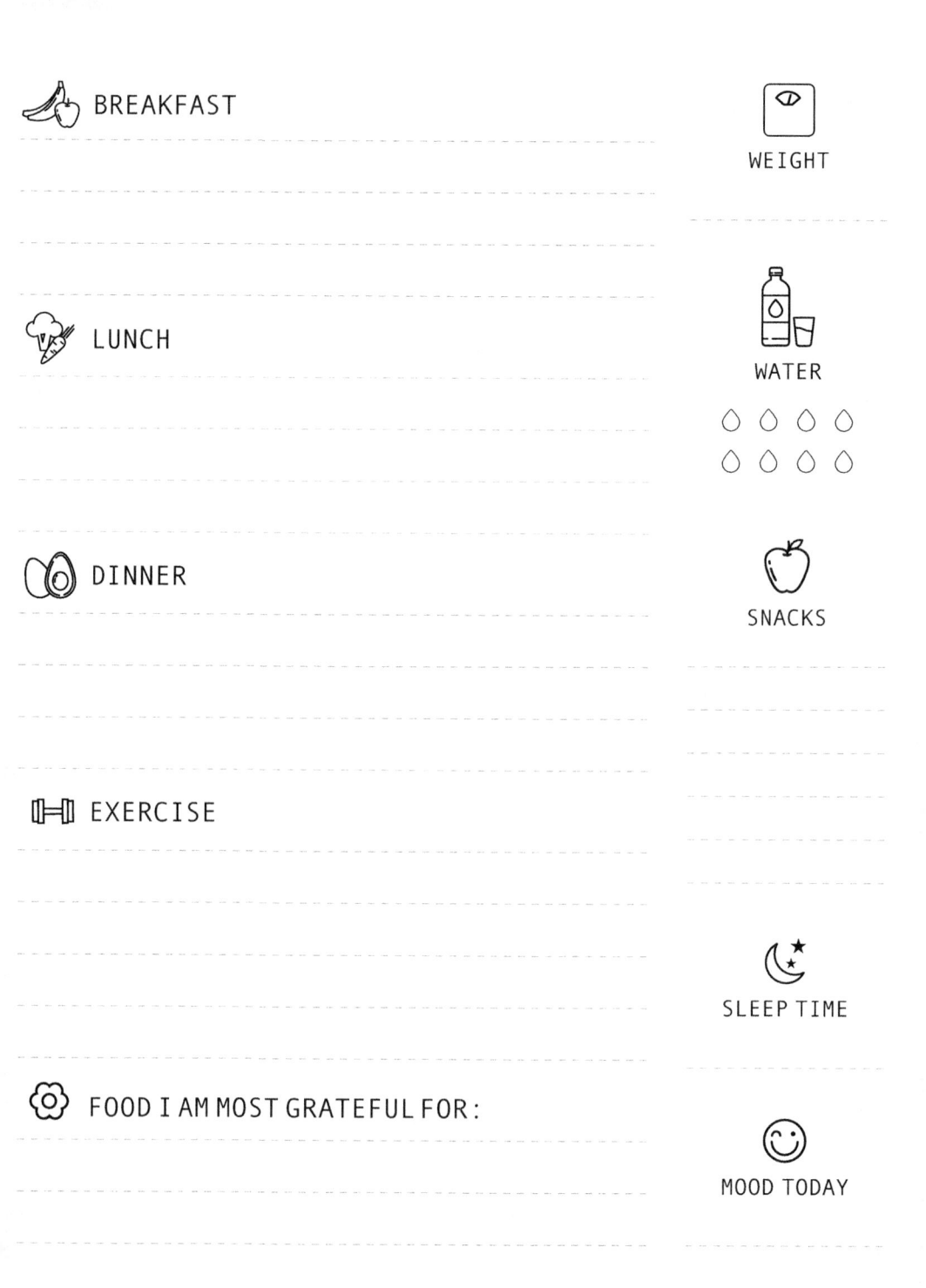

DAY 29

Good things take time.

BREAKFAST

LUNCH

DINNER

EXERCISE

POSITIVE AFFIRMATIONS:

WEIGHT

WATER

○ ○ ○ ○
○ ○ ○ ○

SNACKS

SLEEP TIME

MOOD TODAY

DAY 30

BREAKFAST

WEIGHT

LUNCH

WATER

○ ○ ○ ○
○ ○ ○ ○

DINNER

SNACKS

EXERCISE

SLEEP TIME

MY PROUDEST ACCOMPLISHMENT:

MOOD TODAY

This is me after 30 days

BUST

WAIST

HIPS

THIGH

CALF

WEIGHT

♡ I AM VERY PROUD THAT:

♡ THINGS I'D STILL LIKE TO IMPROVE:

DAY 31

BREAKFAST

WEIGHT

LUNCH

WATER

○ ○ ○ ○
○ ○ ○ ○

DINNER

SNACKS

EXERCISE

SLEEP TIME

ONE ACT OF KINDNESS:

MOOD TODAY

DAY 32   *I can and I will.*

BREAKFAST

LUNCH

DINNER

EXERCISE

MEMORY THAT MAKES ME SMILE:

WEIGHT

WATER

SNACKS

SLEEP TIME

MOOD TODAY

DAY 33

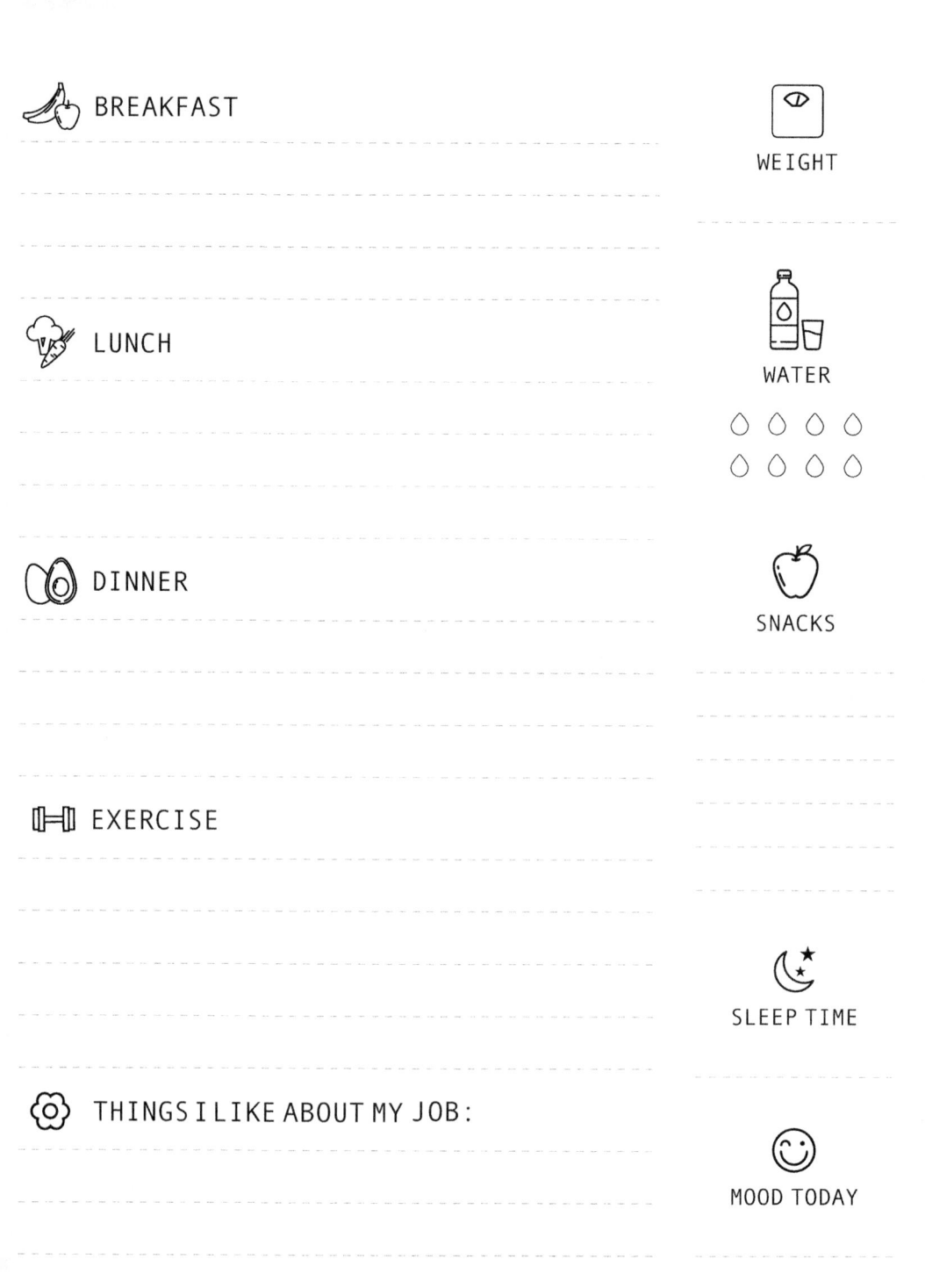

BREAKFAST

WEIGHT

LUNCH

WATER

○ ○ ○ ○
○ ○ ○ ○

DINNER

SNACKS

EXERCISE

SLEEP TIME

THINGS I LIKE ABOUT MY JOB:

MOOD TODAY

DAY 34

BREAKFAST

WEIGHT

LUNCH

WATER

○ ○ ○ ○
○ ○ ○ ○

DINNER

SNACKS

EXERCISE

SLEEP TIME

TODAY'S GOALS:

MOOD TODAY

DAY 35

BREAKFAST

LUNCH

DINNER

EXERCISE

TODAY I AM GRATEFUL FOR:

WEIGHT

WATER

○ ○ ○ ○
○ ○ ○ ○

SNACKS

SLEEP TIME

MOOD TODAY

DAY 36

Don't eat less, just eat right.

BREAKFAST

LUNCH

DINNER

EXERCISE

THINGS TO DO BETTER:

WEIGHT

WATER

○ ○ ○ ○
○ ○ ○ ○

SNACKS

SLEEP TIME

MOOD TODAY

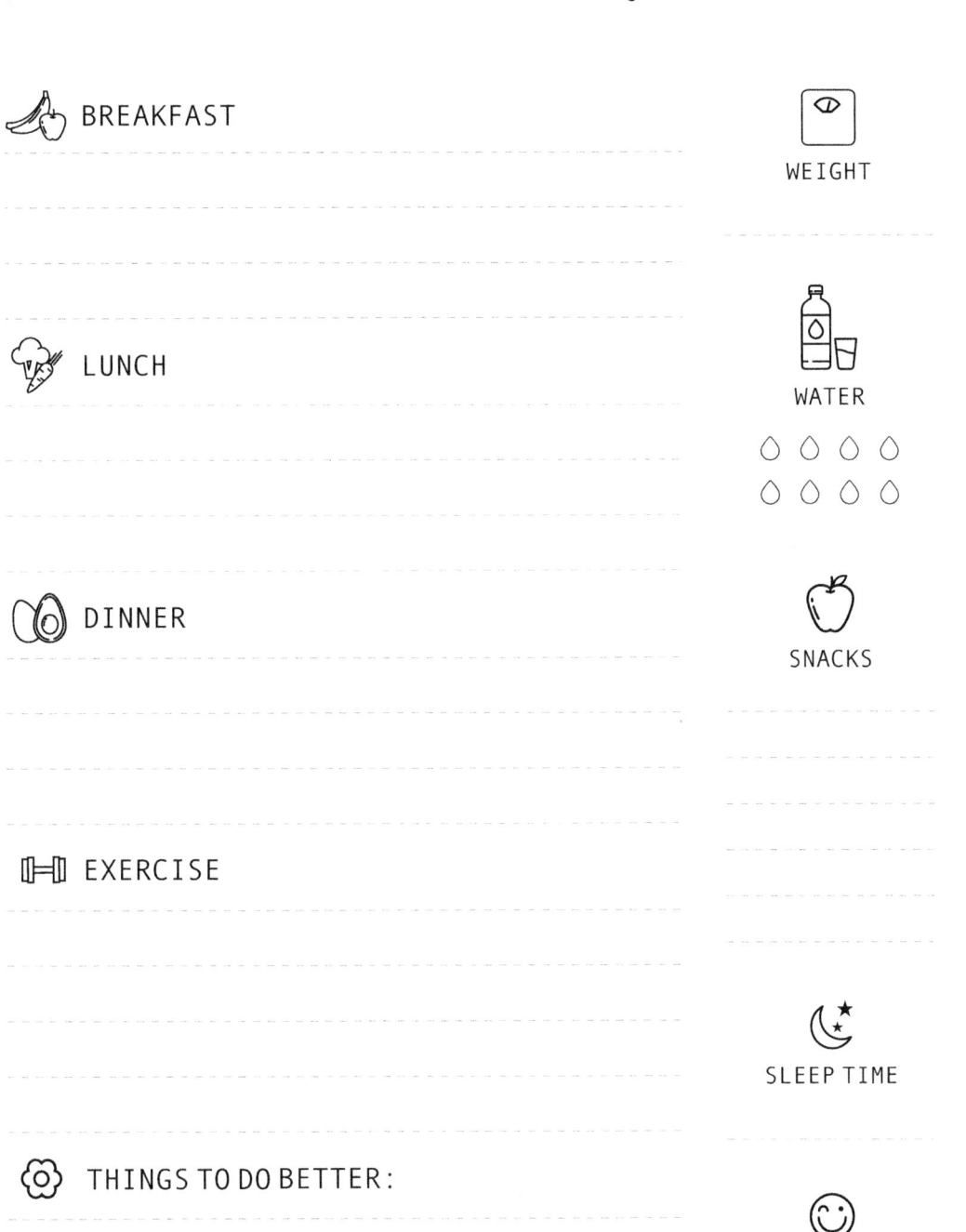

DAY 37

BREAKFAST

WEIGHT

LUNCH

WATER

DINNER

SNACKS

EXERCISE

SLEEP TIME

PEOPLE I AM GRATEFUL FOR:

MOOD TODAY

DAY 38

BREAKFAST

WEIGHT

LUNCH

WATER

○ ○ ○ ○
○ ○ ○ ○

DINNER

SNACKS

EXERCISE

SLEEP TIME

TODAY'S POSITIVE THOUGHTS:

MOOD TODAY

DAY 39

BREAKFAST

WEIGHT

LUNCH

WATER

○ ○ ○ ○
○ ○ ○ ○

DINNER

SNACKS

EXERCISE

SLEEP TIME

A SKILL I AM GRATEFUL FOR:

MOOD TODAY

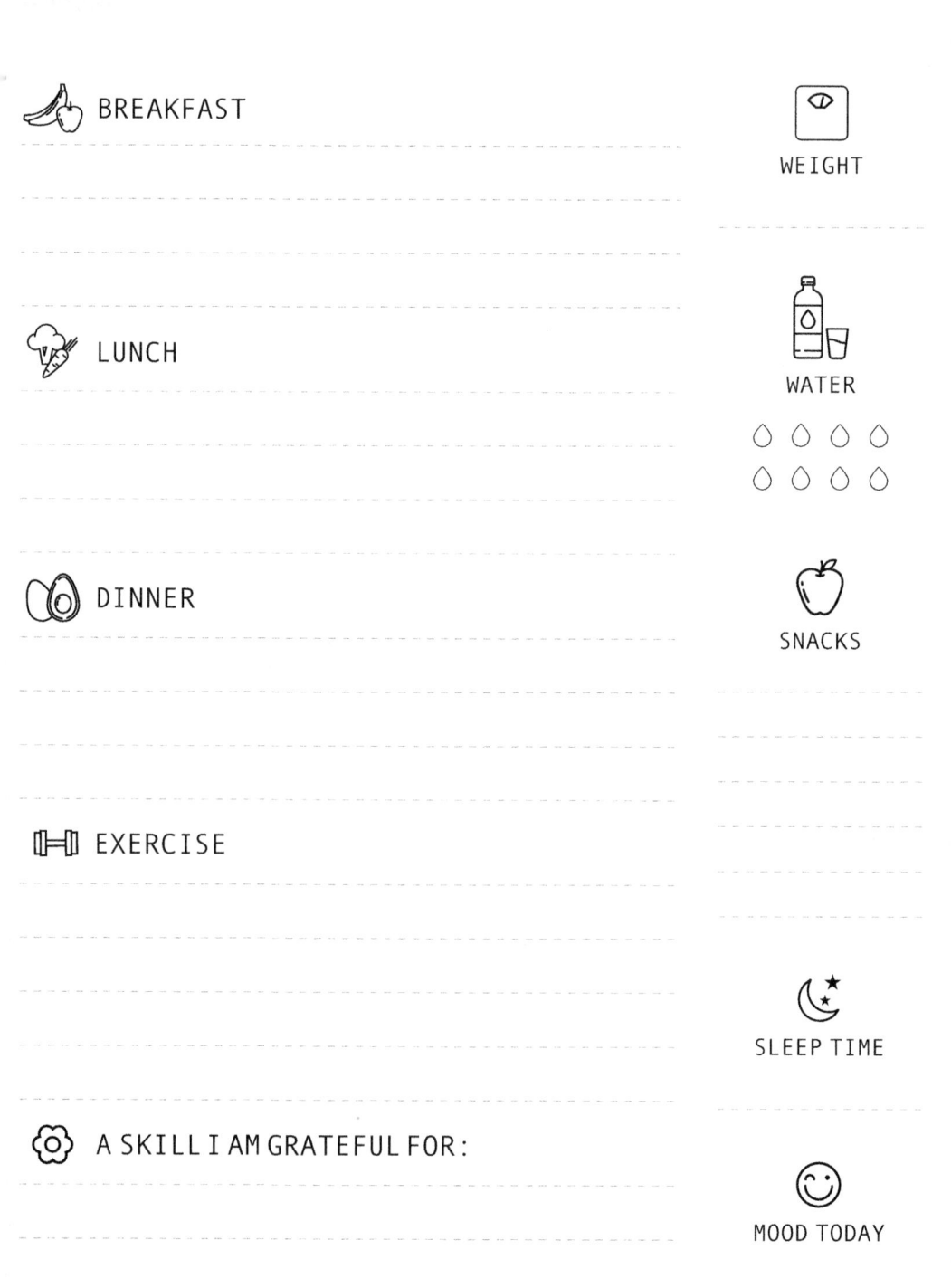

DAY 40

You're gorgeous. Remember that.

BREAKFAST

LUNCH

DINNER

EXERCISE

I WAS KIND TODAY WHEN:

WEIGHT

WATER

○ ○ ○ ○
○ ○ ○ ○

SNACKS

SLEEP TIME

MOOD TODAY

DAY 41

BREAKFAST

LUNCH

DINNER

EXERCISE

ONE ACT OF KINDNESS:

WEIGHT

WATER

SNACKS

SLEEP TIME

MOOD TODAY

DAY 42

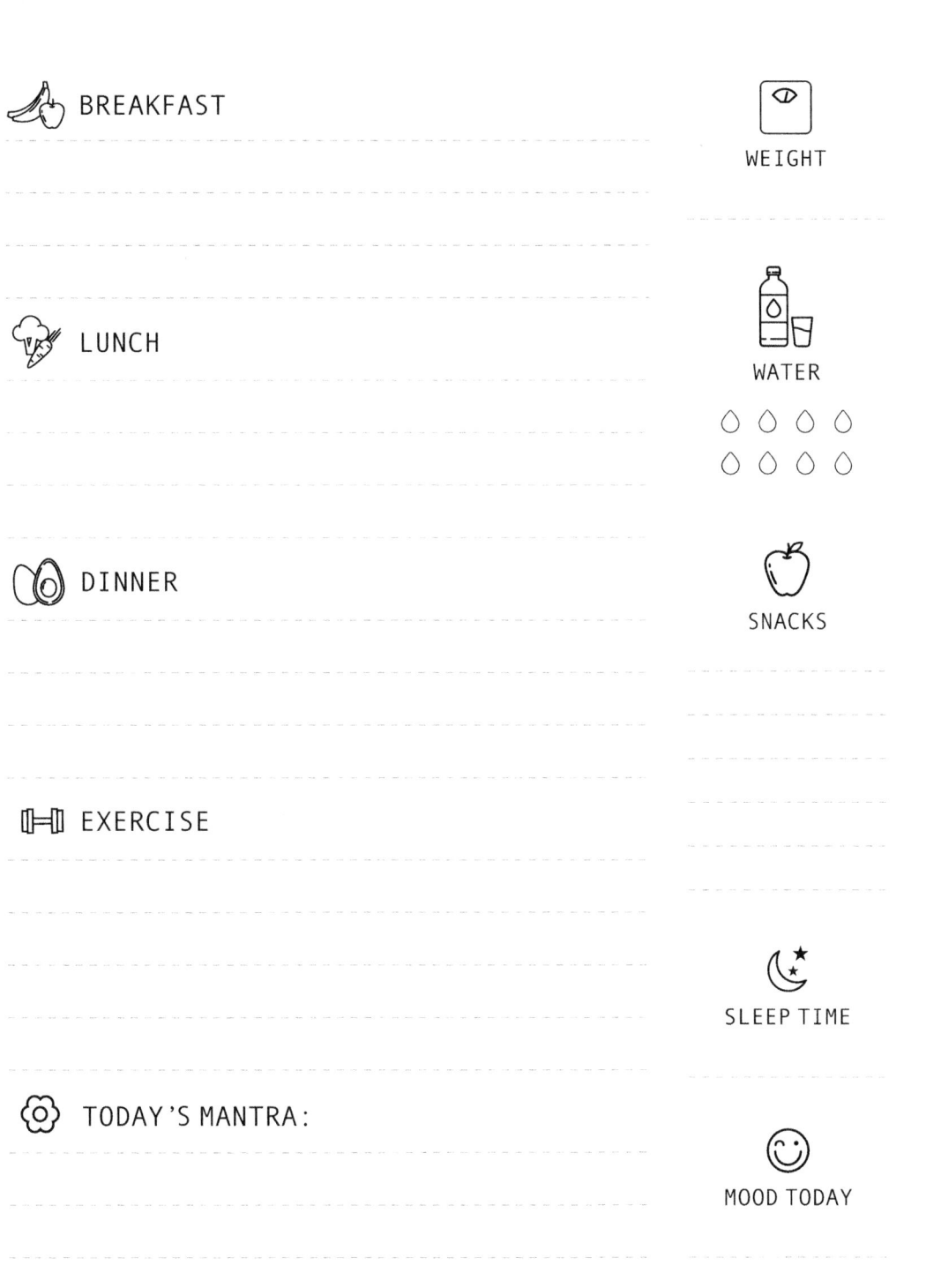

BREAKFAST

WEIGHT

LUNCH

WATER

○ ○ ○ ○
○ ○ ○ ○

DINNER

SNACKS

EXERCISE

SLEEP TIME

TODAY'S MANTRA:

MOOD TODAY

DAY 43

BREAKFAST

LUNCH

DINNER

EXERCISE

THIS INSPIRES ME THE MOST:

WEIGHT

WATER

SNACKS

SLEEP TIME

MOOD TODAY

DAY 44

I'm stronger than my excuses.

BREAKFAST

LUNCH

DINNER

EXERCISE

BEST THING THAT HAPPENED TODAY:

WEIGHT

WATER

○ ○ ○ ○
○ ○ ○ ○

SNACKS

SLEEP TIME

MOOD TODAY

DAY 45

BREAKFAST

LUNCH

DINNER

EXERCISE

MY FAVORITE CHILDOOD MEMORY:

WEIGHT

WATER

SNACKS

SLEEP TIME

MOOD TODAY

DAY 46

BREAKFAST

WEIGHT

LUNCH

WATER

○ ○ ○ ○
○ ○ ○ ○

DINNER

SNACKS

EXERCISE

SLEEP TIME

TODAY'S GOALS:

MOOD TODAY

DAY 47

BREAKFAST

LUNCH

DINNER

EXERCISE

A GOOD THING I DID TODAY:

WEIGHT

WATER

○ ○ ○ ○
○ ○ ○ ○

SNACKS

SLEEP TIME

MOOD TODAY

DAY 48

Keep going.

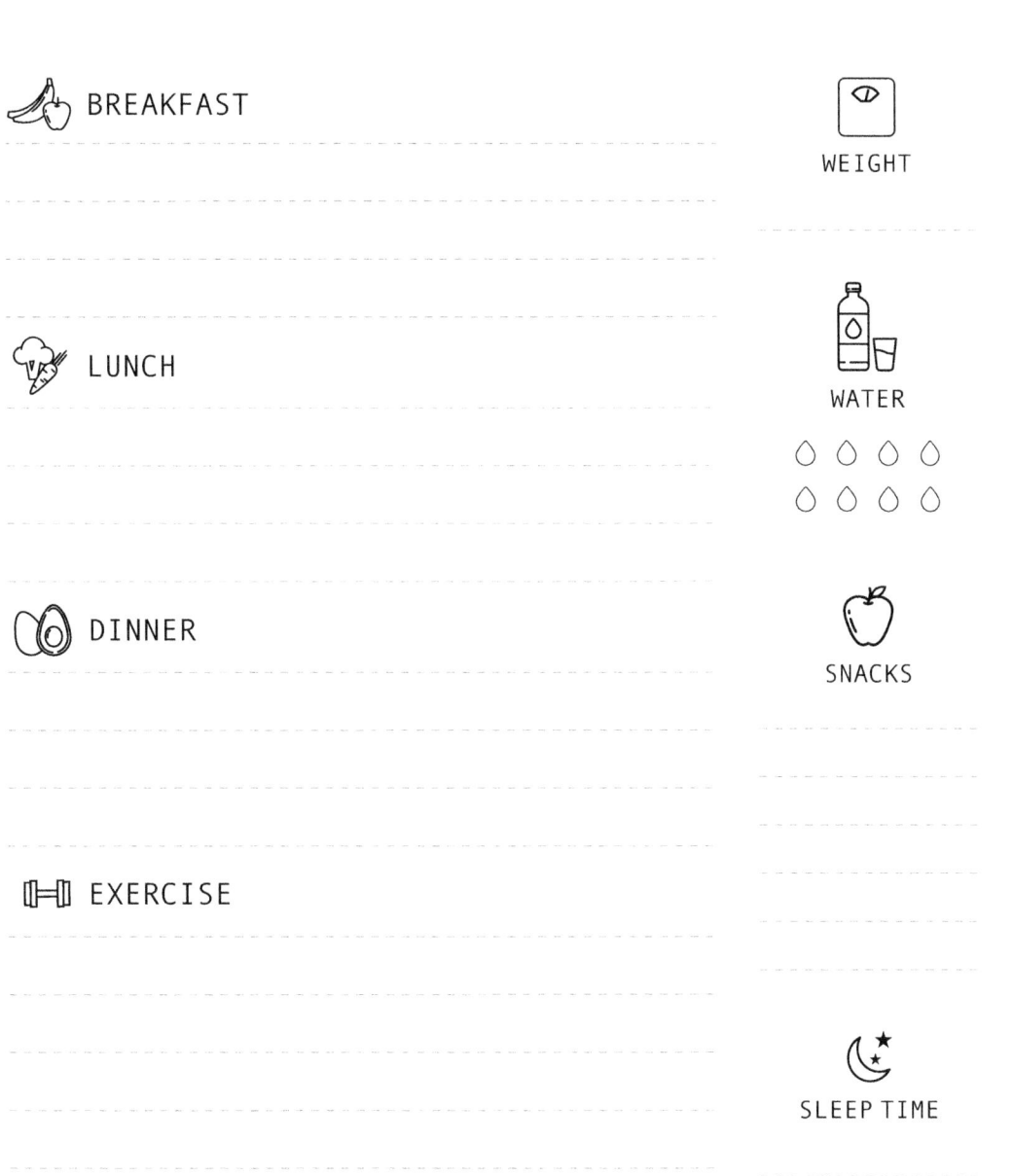

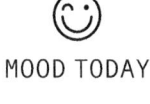

BREAKFAST

WEIGHT

LUNCH

WATER

○ ○ ○ ○
○ ○ ○ ○

DINNER

SNACKS

EXERCISE

SLEEP TIME

THIS MOTIVATES ME:

MOOD TODAY

DAY 49

BREAKFAST

LUNCH

DINNER

EXERCISE

SOMETHING BEAUTIFUL I SAW TODAY:

WEIGHT

WATER

○ ○ ○ ○
○ ○ ○ ○

SNACKS

SLEEP TIME

MOOD TODAY

DAY 50

BREAKFAST

WEIGHT

LUNCH

WATER

○ ○ ○ ○
○ ○ ○ ○

DINNER

SNACKS

EXERCISE

SLEEP TIME

POSITIVE AFFIRMATIONS:

MOOD TODAY

DAY 51

BREAKFAST

WEIGHT

LUNCH

WATER

○ ○ ○ ○
○ ○ ○ ○

DINNER

SNACKS

EXERCISE

SLEEP TIME

COMPLIMENTS I HAVE RECEIVED LATELY:

MOOD TODAY

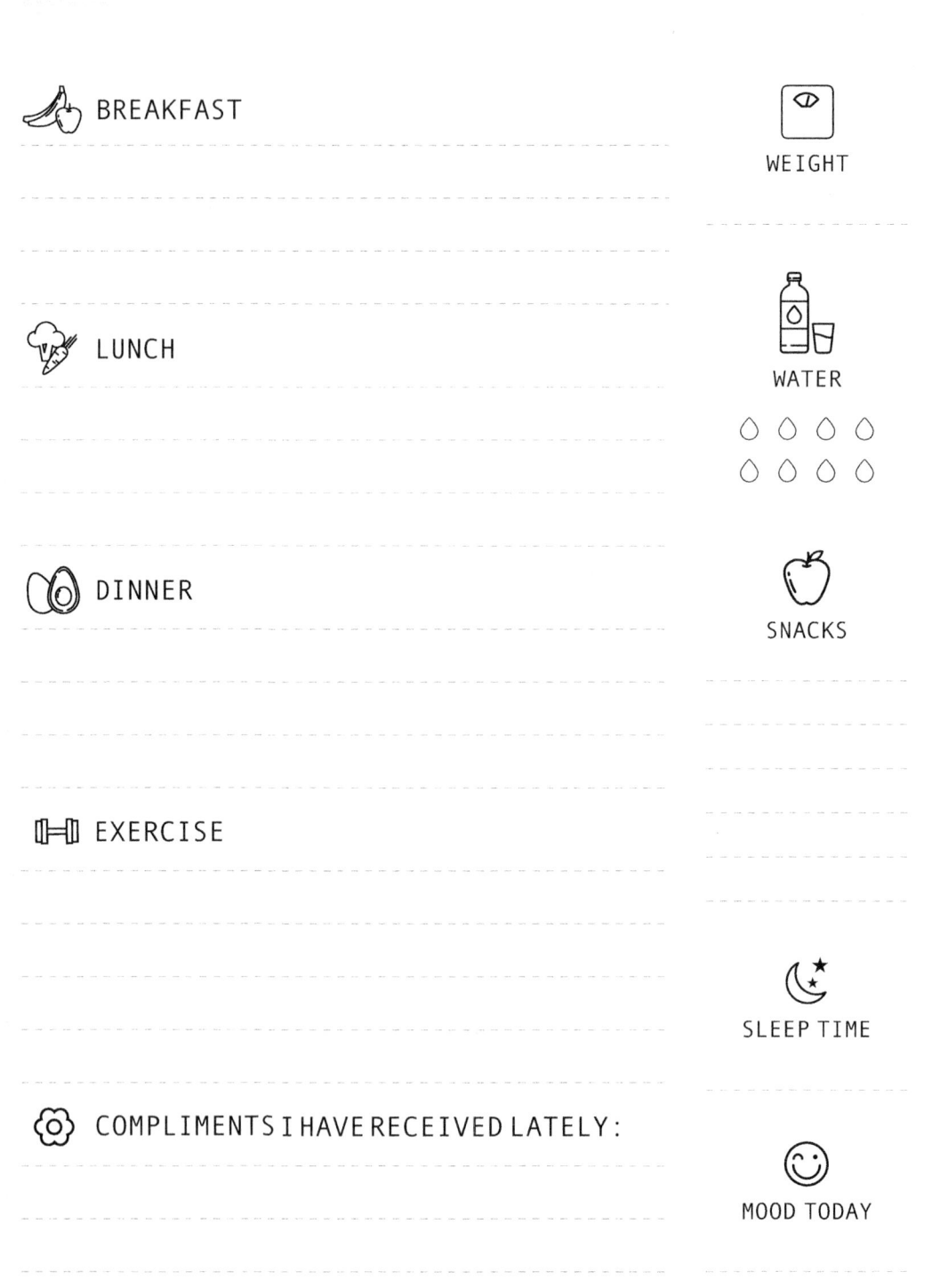

DAY 52

Aim for progress, not perfection.

BREAKFAST

WEIGHT

LUNCH

WATER

○ ○ ○ ○
○ ○ ○ ○

DINNER

SNACKS

EXERCISE

SLEEP TIME

THINGS TO DO BETTER:

MOOD TODAY

DAY 53

BREAKFAST

WEIGHT

LUNCH

WATER

○ ○ ○ ○
○ ○ ○ ○

DINNER

SNACKS

EXERCISE

SLEEP TIME

SMALL THINGS THAT MAKE ME HAPPY:

MOOD TODAY

DAY 54

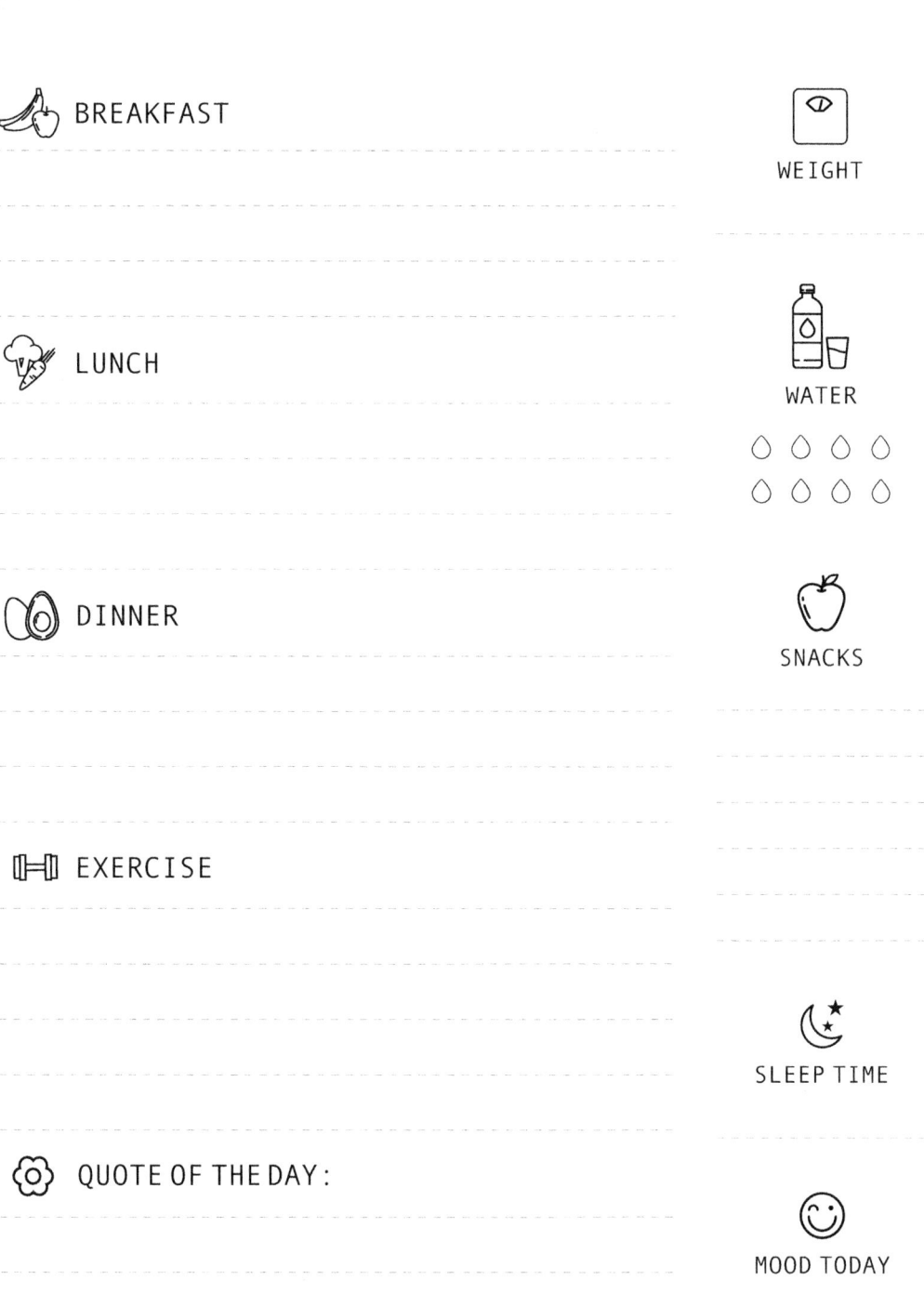

BREAKFAST

WEIGHT

LUNCH

WATER

○ ○ ○ ○
○ ○ ○ ○

DINNER

SNACKS

EXERCISE

SLEEP TIME

QUOTE OF THE DAY:

MOOD TODAY

DAY 55

BREAKFAST

WEIGHT

LUNCH

WATER

○ ○ ○ ○
○ ○ ○ ○

DINNER

SNACKS

EXERCISE

SLEEP TIME

TODAY I AM GRATEFUL FOR:

MOOD TODAY

DAY 56

Positive mind. Positive vibes. Positive life.

BREAKFAST

LUNCH

DINNER

EXERCISE

I LOVE:

WEIGHT

WATER

○ ○ ○ ○
○ ○ ○ ○

SNACKS

SLEEP TIME

MOOD TODAY

DAY 57

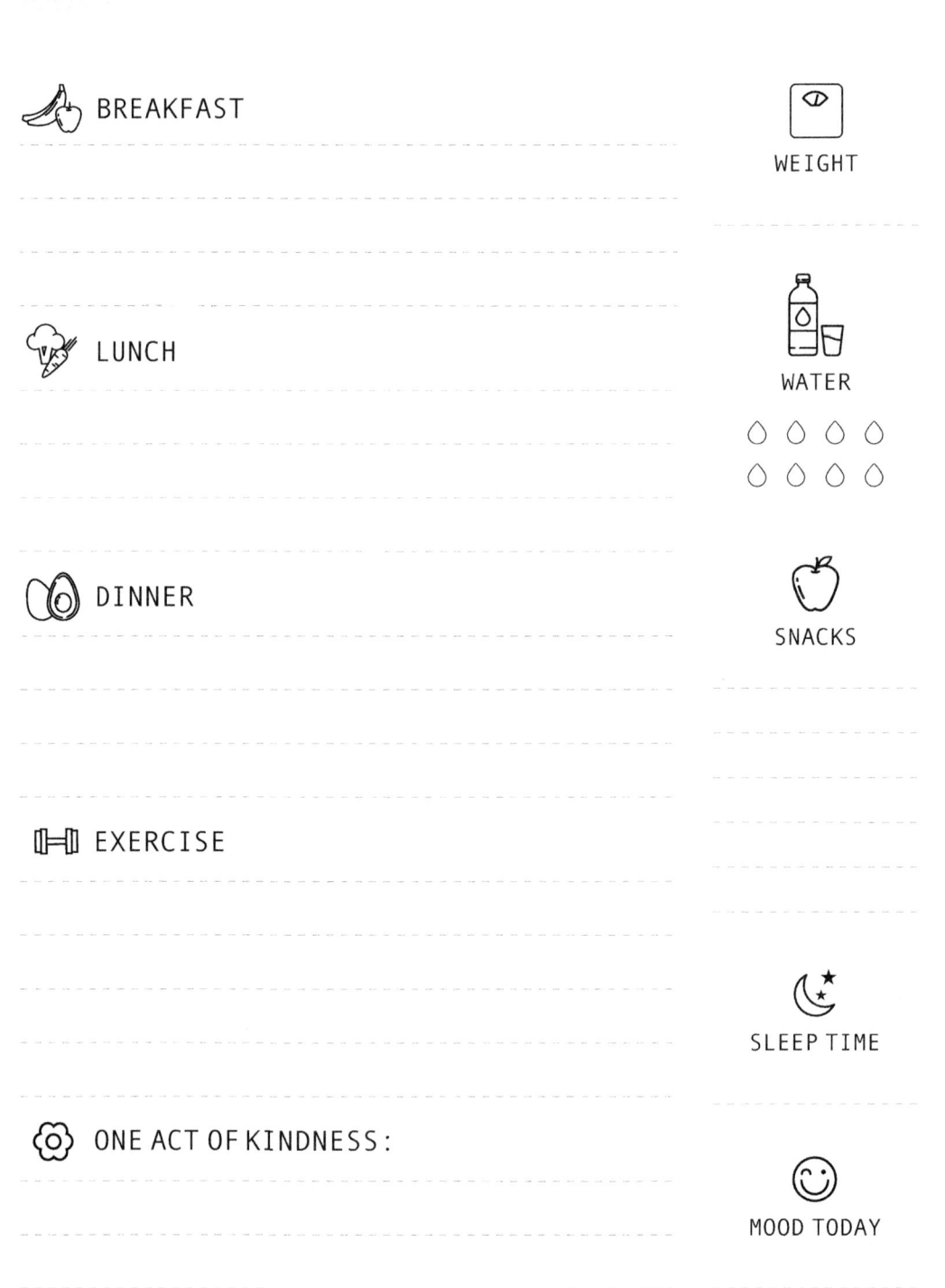

BREAKFAST

WEIGHT

LUNCH

WATER

○ ○ ○ ○
○ ○ ○ ○

DINNER

SNACKS

EXERCISE

SLEEP TIME

ONE ACT OF KINDNESS:

MOOD TODAY

DAY 58

BREAKFAST

WEIGHT

LUNCH

WATER

○ ○ ○ ○
○ ○ ○ ○

DINNER

SNACKS

EXERCISE

SLEEP TIME

TODAY'S MANTRA:

MOOD TODAY

DAY 59

🍌 BREAKFAST

🥗 LUNCH

🥑 DINNER

🏋 EXERCISE

🌼 THINGS THAT MAKE ME HAPPY:

WEIGHT

WATER
○ ○ ○ ○
○ ○ ○ ○

SNACKS

SLEEP TIME

MOOD TODAY

DAY 60

good food = good mood.

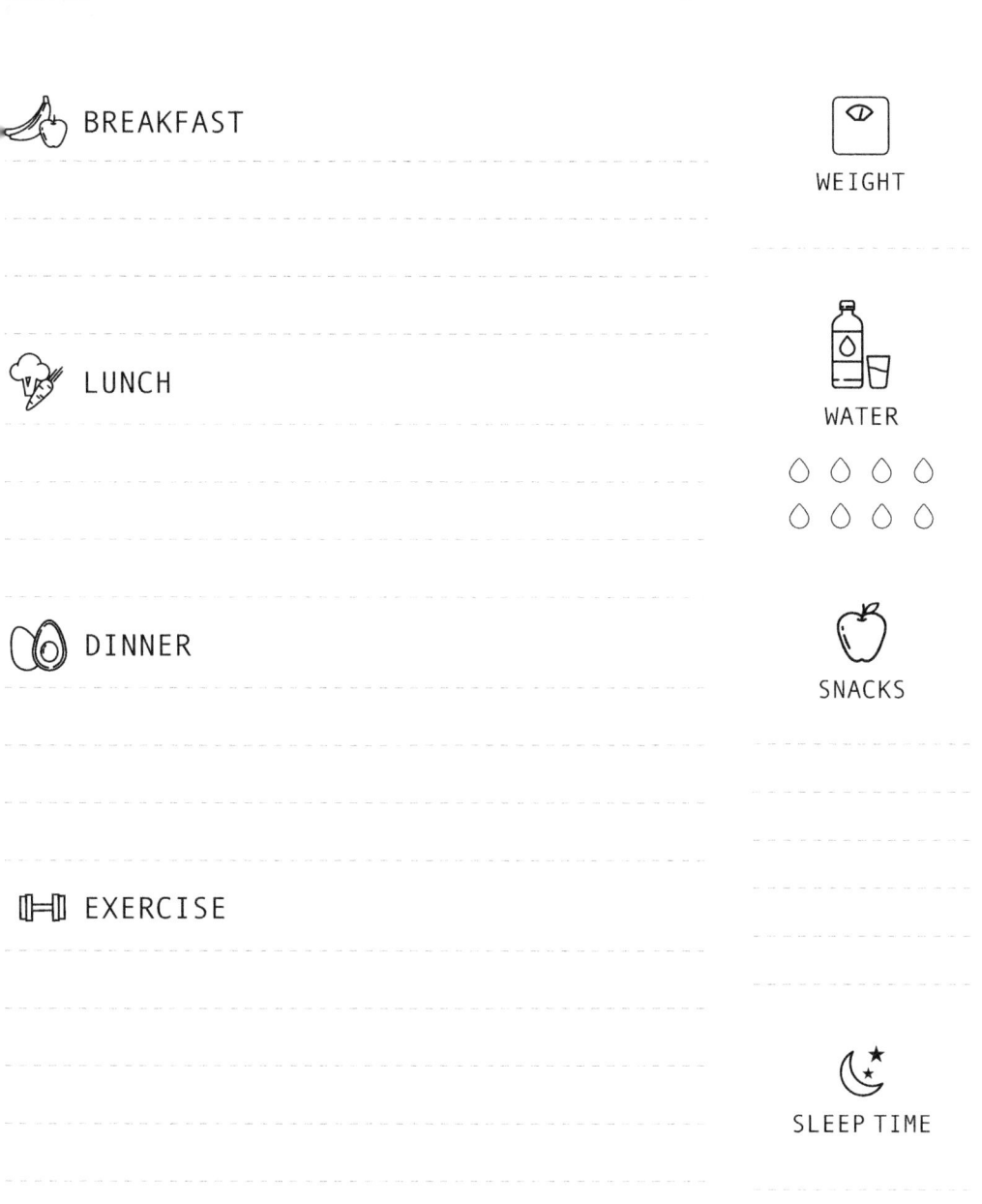

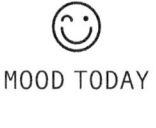

BREAKFAST

LUNCH

DINNER

EXERCISE

A CHALLENGE I AM GRATEFUL FOR:

WEIGHT

WATER
○ ○ ○ ○
○ ○ ○ ○

SNACKS

SLEEP TIME

MOOD TODAY

This is me after 60 days

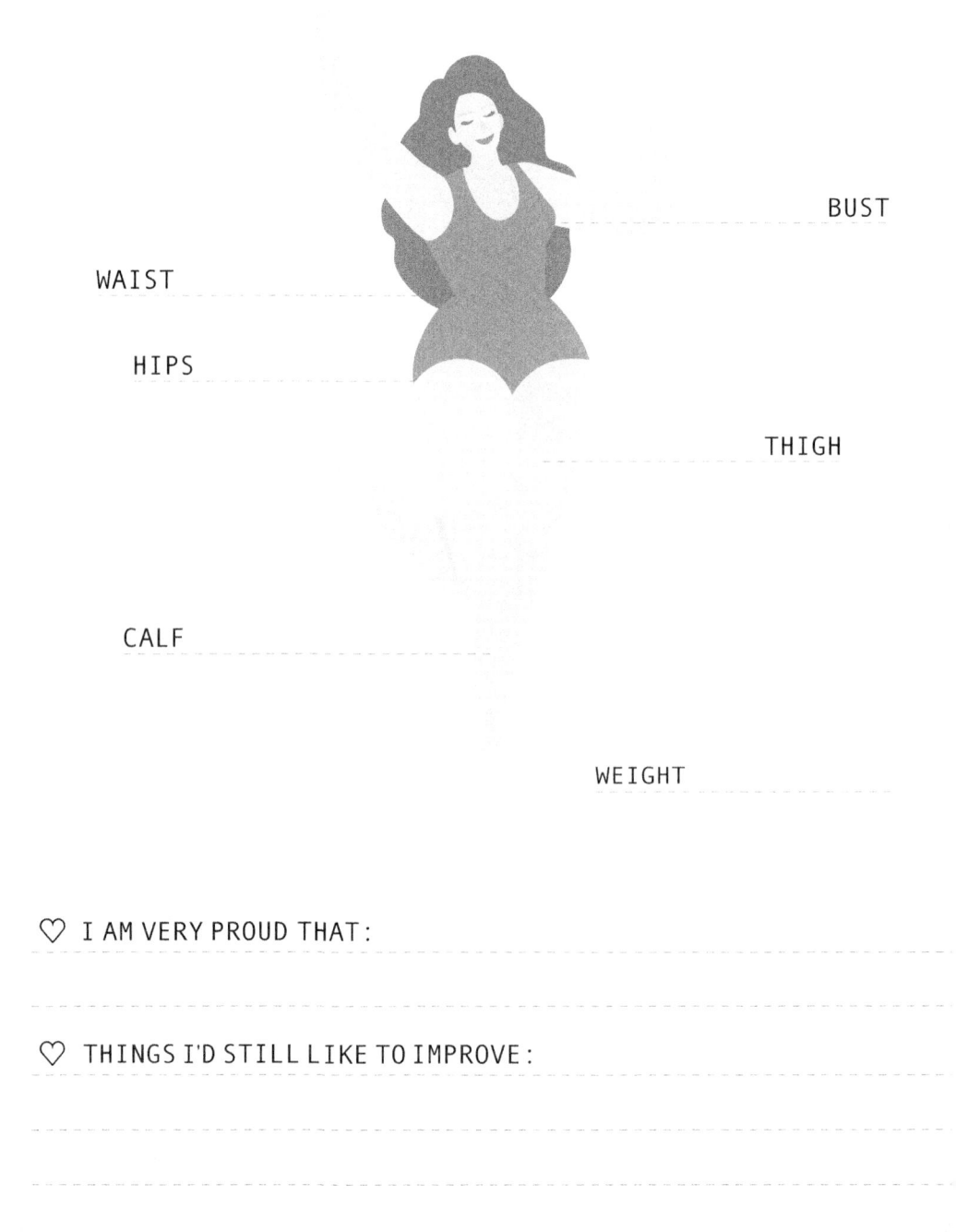

BUST

WAIST

HIPS

THIGH

CALF

WEIGHT

♡ I AM VERY PROUD THAT :

♡ THINGS I'D STILL LIKE TO IMPROVE :

DAY 61

BREAKFAST

LUNCH

DINNER

EXERCISE

TODAY'S GOALS:

WEIGHT

WATER

SNACKS

SLEEP TIME

MOOD TODAY

DAY 62

🍌 BREAKFAST

⚖️ WEIGHT

🥦 LUNCH

💧 WATER

○ ○ ○ ○
○ ○ ○ ○

🥑 DINNER

🍎 SNACKS

🏋️ EXERCISE

🌙 SLEEP TIME

🌼 A GOOD THING I DID TODAY:

☺️ MOOD TODAY

DAY 63

Slow progress is still progress.

BREAKFAST

LUNCH

DINNER

EXERCISE

TODAY I WAS HELPFUL WHEN:

WEIGHT

WATER

○ ○ ○ ○
○ ○ ○ ○

SNACKS

SLEEP TIME

MOOD TODAY

DAY 64

BREAKFAST

LUNCH

DINNER

EXERCISE

POSITIVE PEOPLE IN MY LIFE:

WEIGHT

WATER

○ ○ ○ ○
○ ○ ○ ○

SNACKS

SLEEP TIME

MOOD TODAY

DAY 65

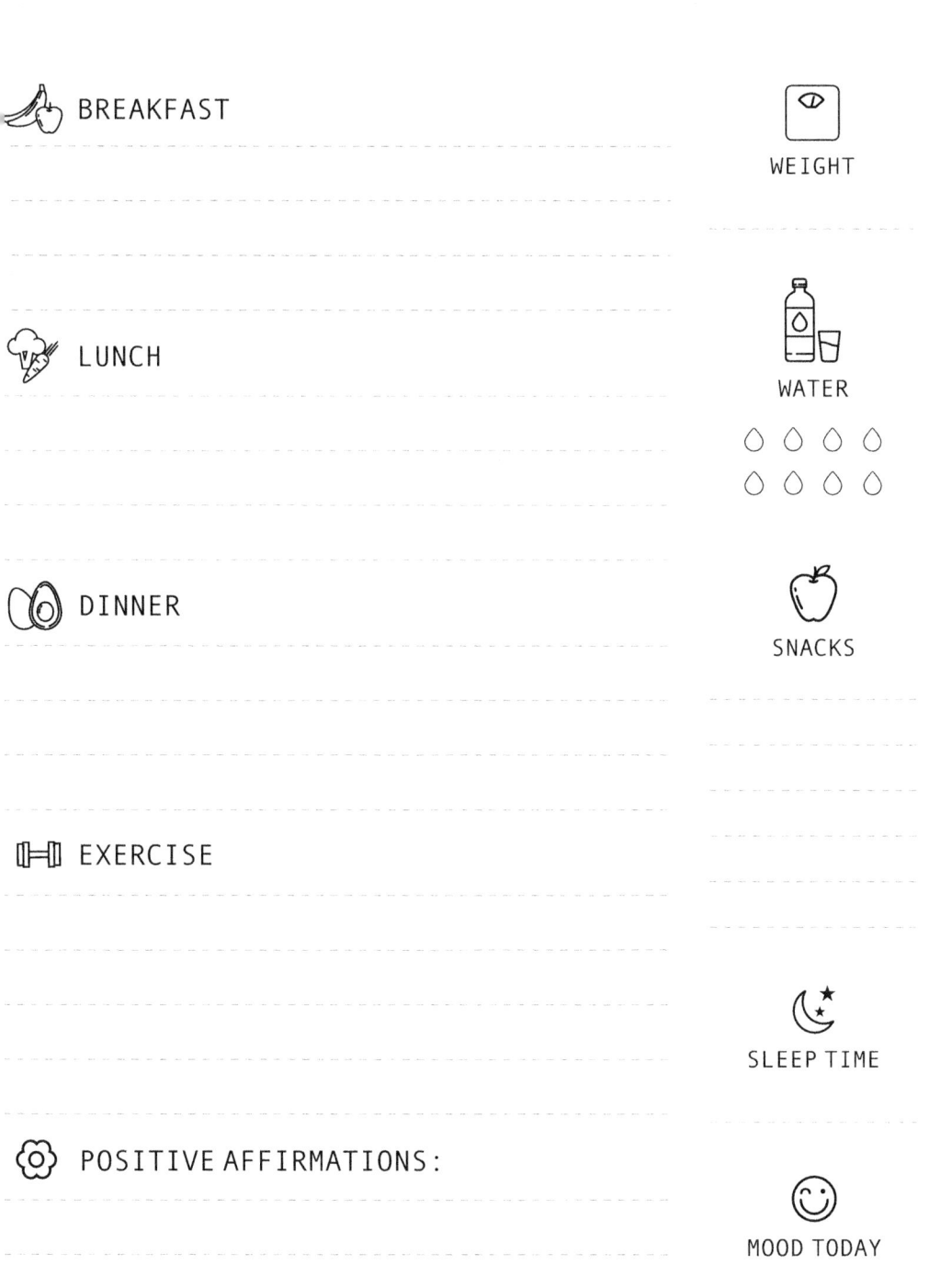

BREAKFAST

WEIGHT

LUNCH

WATER

DINNER

SNACKS

EXERCISE

SLEEP TIME

POSITIVE AFFIRMATIONS:

MOOD TODAY

DAY 66

BREAKFAST

WEIGHT

LUNCH

WATER

○ ○ ○ ○
○ ○ ○ ○

DINNER

SNACKS

EXERCISE

SLEEP TIME

THINGS THAT MADE ME SMILE TODAY:

MOOD TODAY

DAY 67

Less comparison, more compassion.

BREAKFAST

WEIGHT

LUNCH

WATER

○ ○ ○ ○
○ ○ ○ ○

DINNER

SNACKS

EXERCISE

SLEEP TIME

THINGS I AM PROUD OF MYSELF FOR:

MOOD TODAY

DAY 68

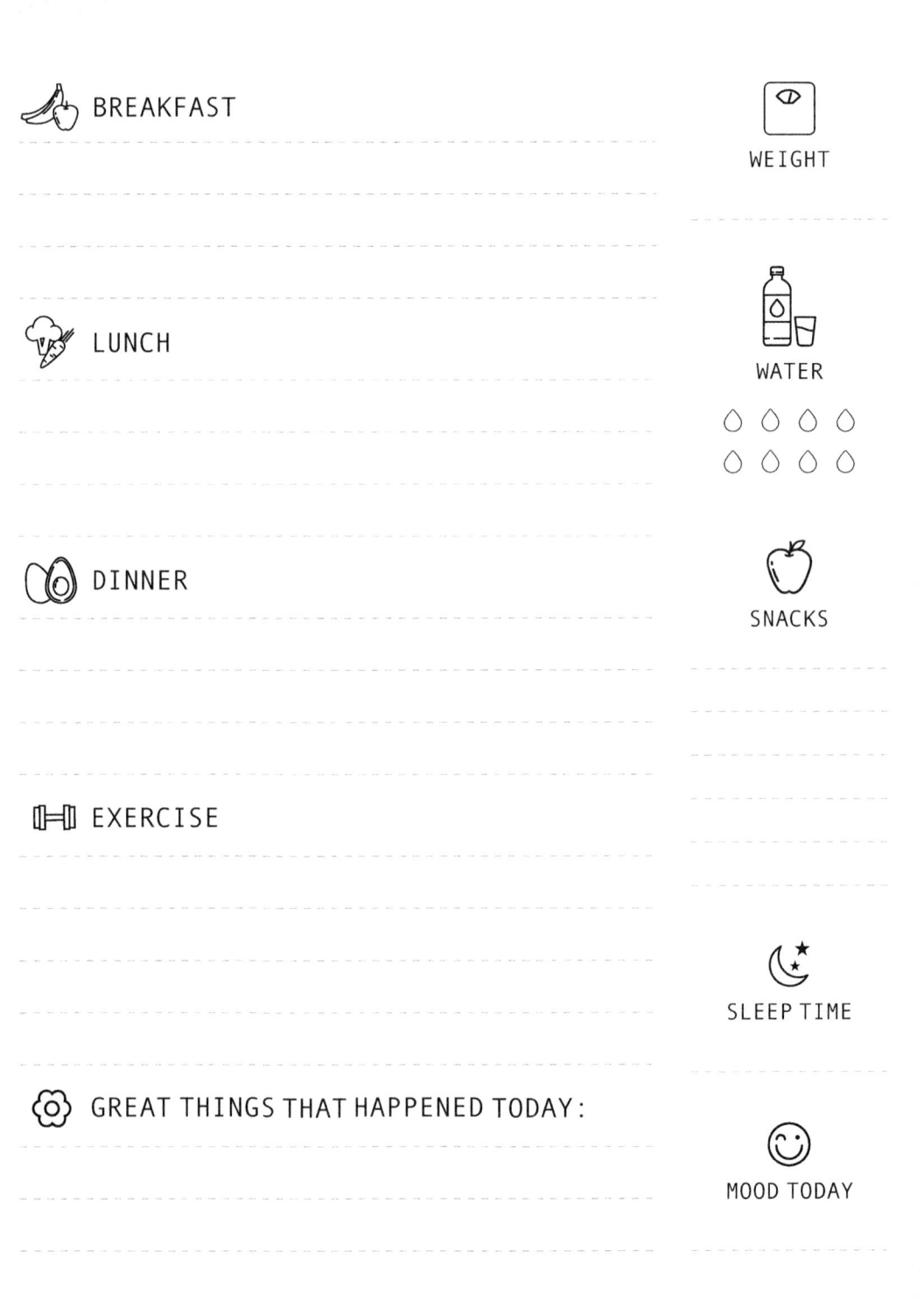

BREAKFAST

WEIGHT

LUNCH

WATER

DINNER

SNACKS

EXERCISE

SLEEP TIME

GREAT THINGS THAT HAPPENED TODAY:

MOOD TODAY

DAY 69

BREAKFAST

WEIGHT

LUNCH

WATER

○ ○ ○ ○
○ ○ ○ ○

DINNER

SNACKS

EXERCISE

SLEEP TIME

MY GOALS FOR TOMORROW:

MOOD TODAY

DAY 70

BREAKFAST

LUNCH

DINNER

EXERCISE

I CHOOSE TO LOVE MYSELF BECAUSE:

WEIGHT

WATER

SNACKS

SLEEP TIME

MOOD TODAY

DAY 71

Remember why you started.

🍌 BREAKFAST

WEIGHT

🥦 LUNCH

WATER

○ ○ ○ ○
○ ○ ○ ○

🥑 DINNER

SNACKS

🏋 EXERCISE

SLEEP TIME

❀ I WAS AWESOME TODAY BECAUSE:

MOOD TODAY

DAY 72

BREAKFAST

LUNCH

DINNER

EXERCISE

ONE ACT OF KINDNESS:

WEIGHT

WATER

SNACKS

SLEEP TIME

MOOD TODAY

DAY 73

BREAKFAST

LUNCH

DINNER

EXERCISE

TODAY'S MANTRA:

WEIGHT

WATER

SNACKS

SLEEP TIME

MOOD TODAY

DAY 74

BREAKFAST

WEIGHT

LUNCH

WATER

DINNER

SNACKS

EXERCISE

SLEEP TIME

POSITIVE EMOTIONS EXPERIENCED TODAY:

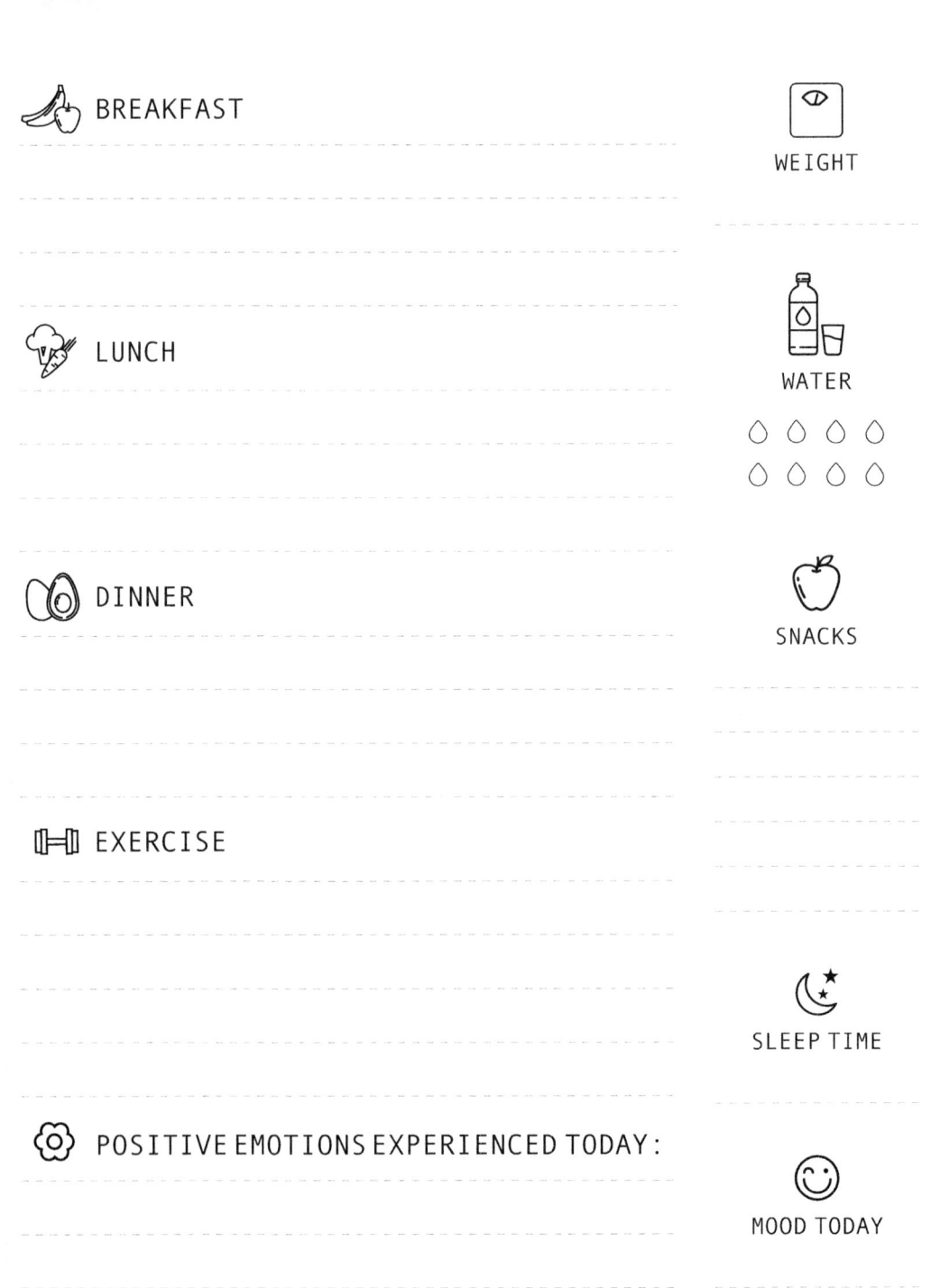

MOOD TODAY

DAY 75

See good in all things.

BREAKFAST

LUNCH

DINNER

EXERCISE

MY FAVORITE QUOTE:

WEIGHT

WATER

SNACKS

SLEEP TIME

MOOD TODAY

DAY 76

BREAKFAST

WEIGHT

LUNCH

WATER

○ ○ ○ ○
○ ○ ○ ○

DINNER

SNACKS

EXERCISE

SLEEP TIME

I FELT GOOD ABOUT MYSELF WHEN:

MOOD TODAY

DAY 77

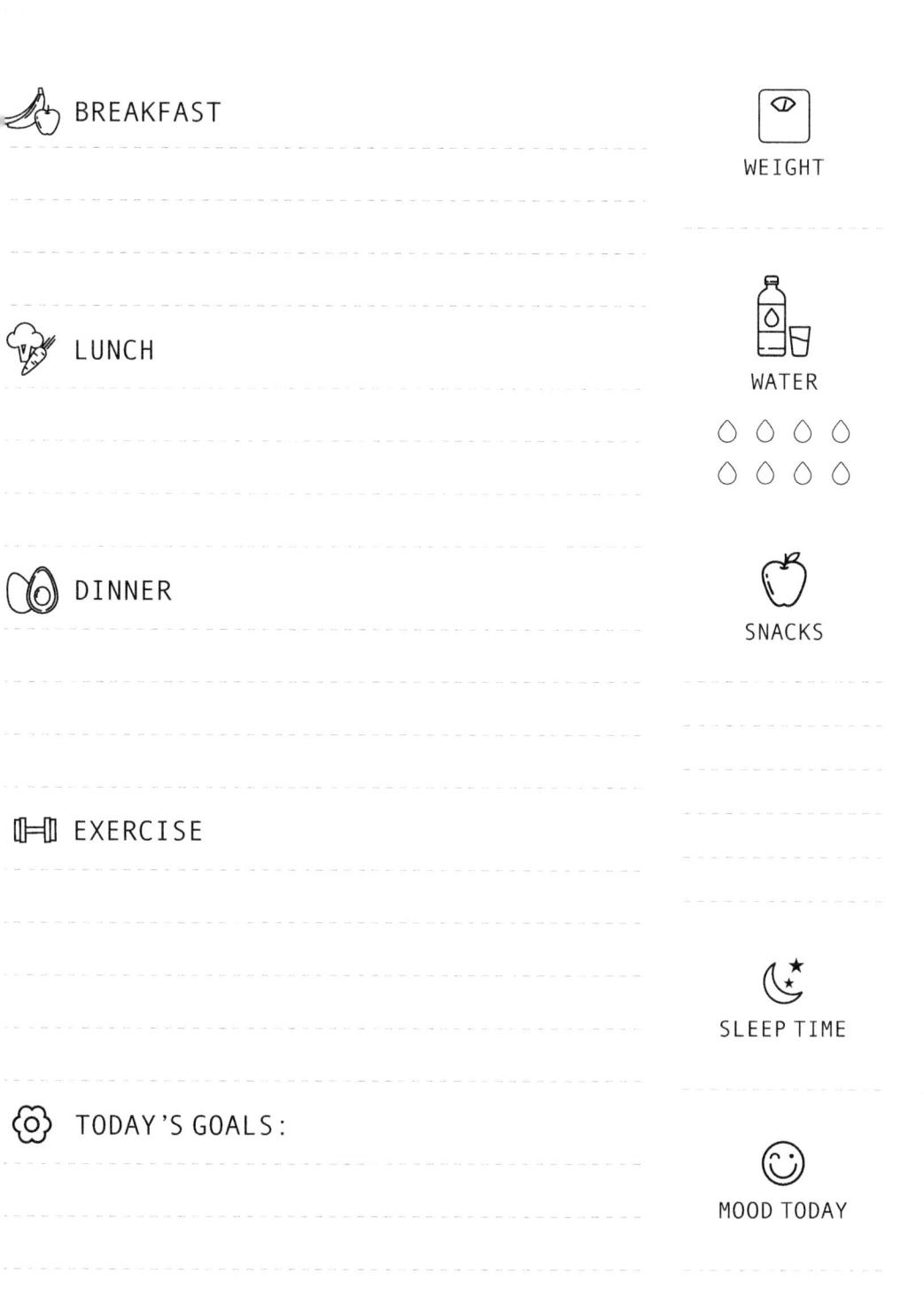

🍌 BREAKFAST

WEIGHT

🥦 LUNCH

WATER

○ ○ ○ ○
○ ○ ○ ○

🥑 DINNER

SNACKS

🏋 EXERCISE

SLEEP TIME

❀ TODAY'S GOALS:

MOOD TODAY

DAY 78

BREAKFAST

WEIGHT

LUNCH

WATER

DINNER

SNACKS

EXERCISE

SLEEP TIME

A GOOD THING I DID TODAY:

MOOD TODAY

DAY 79

Focus on your health, not your weight.

BREAKFAST

LUNCH

DINNER

EXERCISE

SOMETHING BEAUTIFUL I AM THANKFUL FOR:

WEIGHT

WATER

○ ○ ○ ○
○ ○ ○ ○

SNACKS

SLEEP TIME

MOOD TODAY

DAY 80

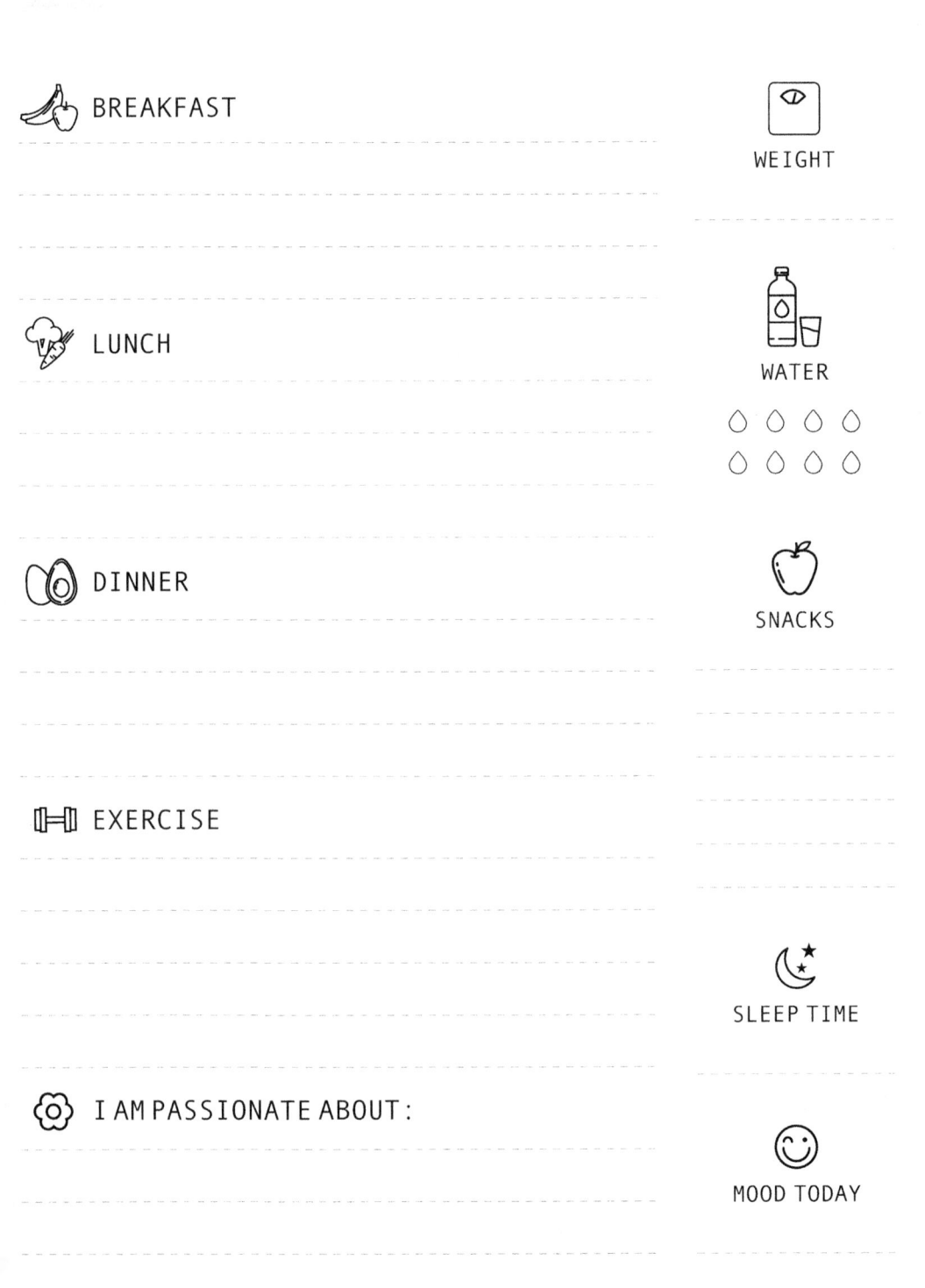

BREAKFAST

LUNCH

DINNER

EXERCISE

I AM PASSIONATE ABOUT:

WEIGHT

WATER

SNACKS

SLEEP TIME

MOOD TODAY

DAY 81

🍌 BREAKFAST

WEIGHT

🥦 LUNCH

WATER

○ ○ ○ ○
○ ○ ○ ○

🥑 DINNER

SNACKS

🏋 EXERCISE

SLEEP TIME

🌸 POSITIVE AFFIRMATIONS:

MOOD TODAY

DAY 82

BREAKFAST

LUNCH

DINNER

EXERCISE

POSITIVE THINGS ABOUT MY LIFE:

WEIGHT

WATER

SNACKS

SLEEP TIME

MOOD TODAY

DAY 83

Rise and shine.

BREAKFAST

WEIGHT

LUNCH

WATER

○ ○ ○ ○
○ ○ ○ ○

DINNER

SNACKS

EXERCISE

SLEEP TIME

I AM REALLY GOOD AT:

MOOD TODAY

DAY 84

BREAKFAST

WEIGHT

LUNCH

WATER

○ ○ ○ ○
○ ○ ○ ○

DINNER

SNACKS

EXERCISE

SLEEP TIME

I WANT PEOPLE TO THINK OF ME AS:

MOOD TODAY

DAY 85

BREAKFAST

WEIGHT

LUNCH

WATER

○ ○ ○ ○
○ ○ ○ ○

DINNER

SNACKS

EXERCISE

SLEEP TIME

TODAY'S POSITIVE THOUGHTS:

MOOD TODAY

DAY 86

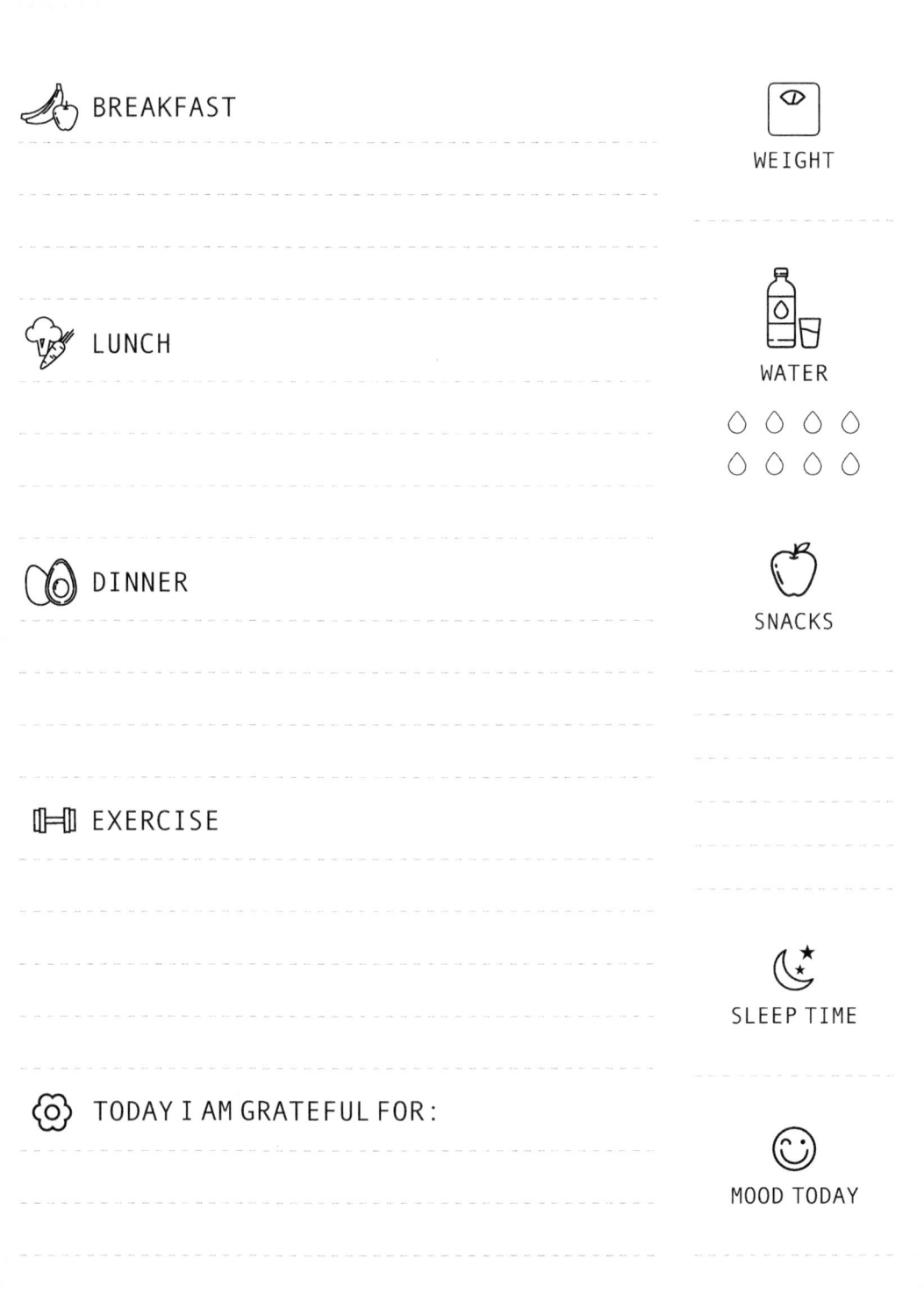

🍌 **BREAKFAST**

🥕 **LUNCH**

🥑 **DINNER**

🏋 **EXERCISE**

🌸 **TODAY I AM GRATEFUL FOR:**

WEIGHT

WATER
○ ○ ○ ○
○ ○ ○ ○

SNACKS

SLEEP TIME

MOOD TODAY

DAY 87

Don't stop until you're proud.

BREAKFAST

WEIGHT

LUNCH

WATER

○ ○ ○ ○
○ ○ ○ ○

DINNER

SNACKS

EXERCISE

SLEEP TIME

THE PERSON I AM MOST THANKFUL FOR:

MOOD TODAY

DAY 88

BREAKFAST

WEIGHT

LUNCH

WATER

○ ○ ○ ○
○ ○ ○ ○

DINNER

SNACKS

EXERCISE

SLEEP TIME

ONE ACT OF KINDNESS :

MOOD TODAY

DAY 89

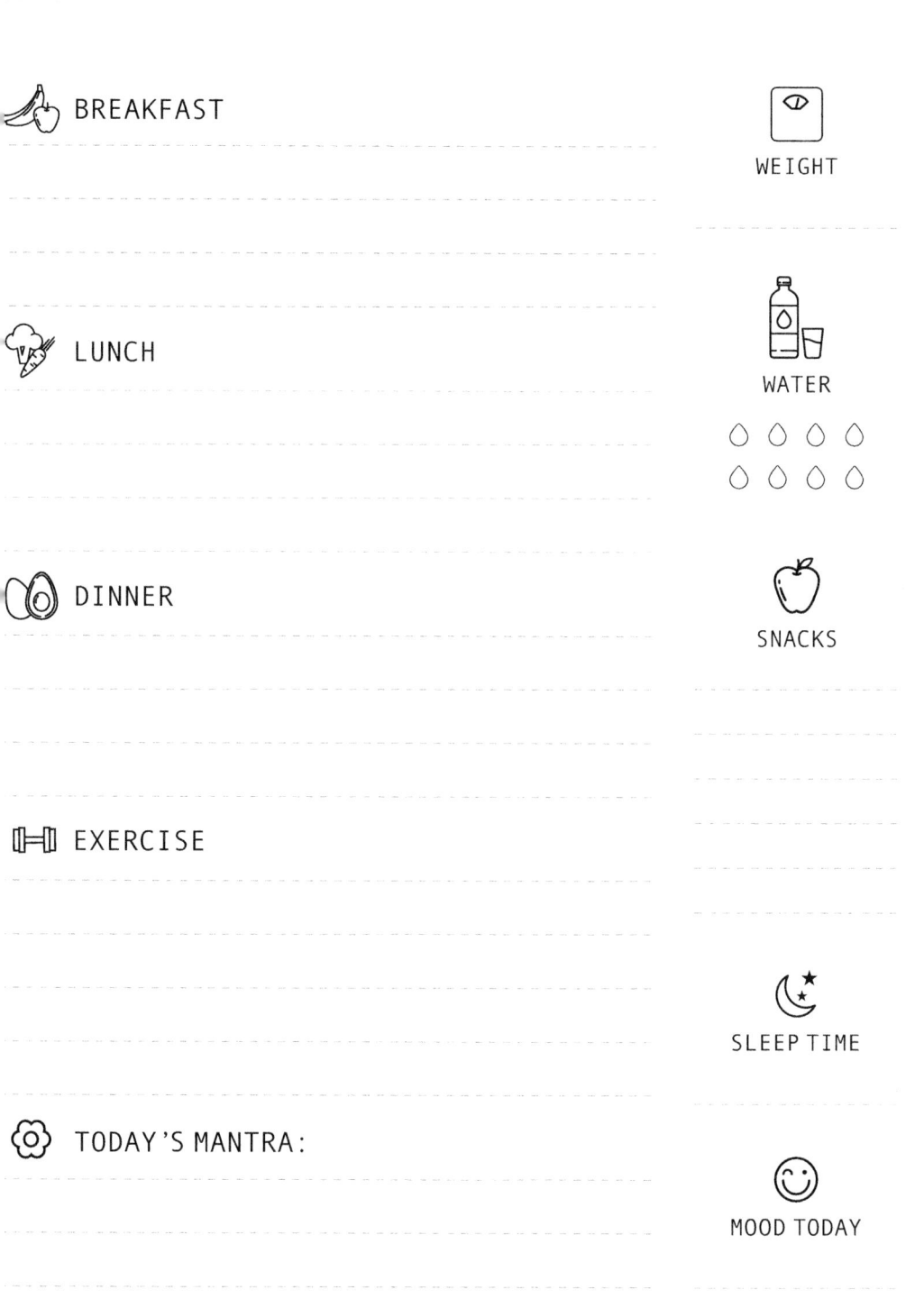

🍌 BREAKFAST

WEIGHT

🥦 LUNCH

WATER

💧 💧 💧 💧
💧 💧 💧 💧

🥑 DINNER

🍎 SNACKS

🏋 EXERCISE

🌙 SLEEP TIME

🌼 TODAY'S MANTRA:

☺ MOOD TODAY

DAY 90

BREAKFAST

WEIGHT

LUNCH

WATER

○ ○ ○ ○
○ ○ ○ ○

DINNER

SNACKS

EXERCISE

SLEEP TIME

A LONG TERM GOAL I HAVE IS:

MOOD TODAY

This is me after 90 days

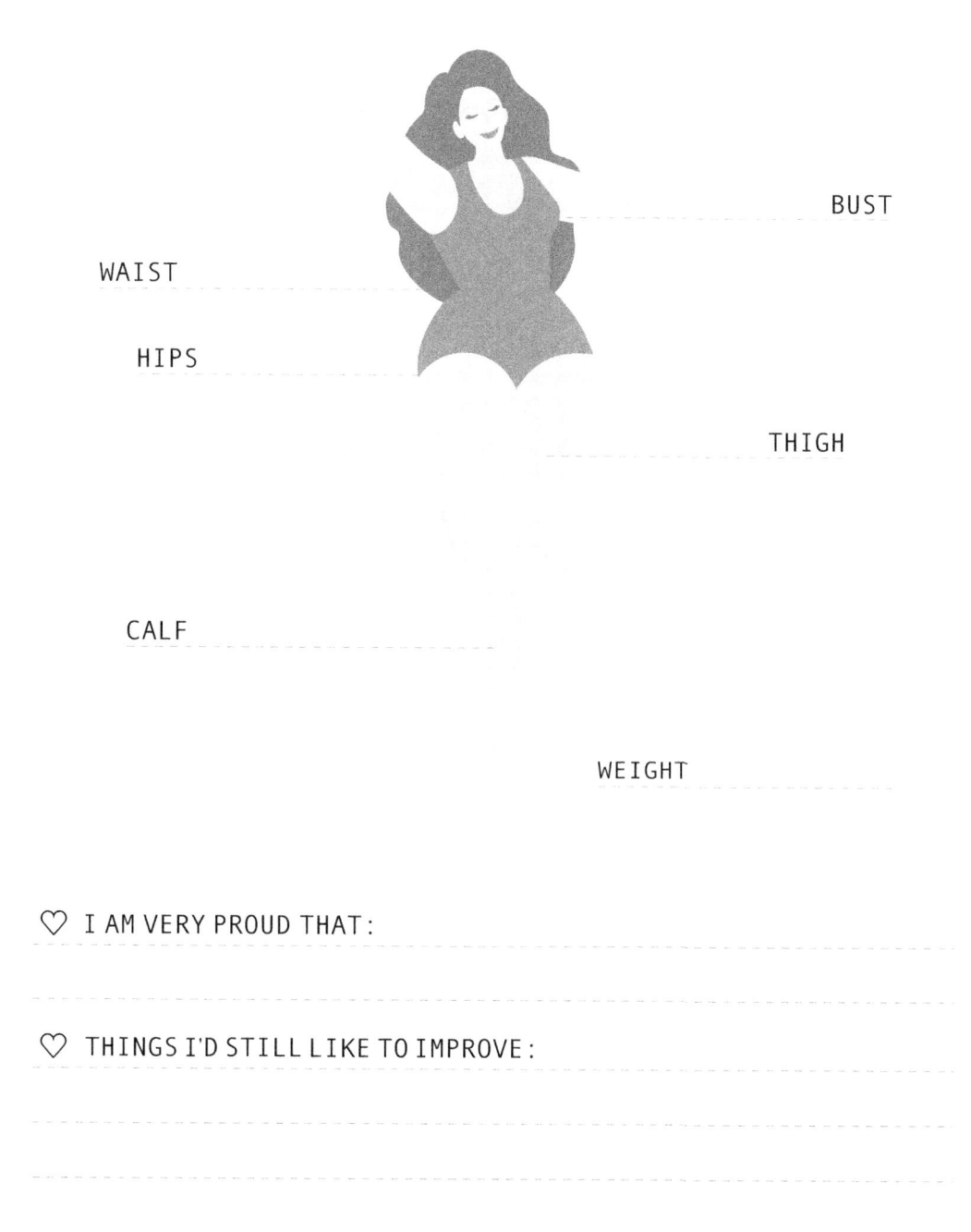

BUST

WAIST

HIPS

THIGH

CALF

WEIGHT

♡ I AM VERY PROUD THAT :

♡ THINGS I'D STILL LIKE TO IMPROVE :

30-day challenge

DAY 1	DAY 2	DAY 3
DAY 4	DAY 5	DAY 6
DAY 7	DAY 8	DAY 9
DAY 10	DAY 11	DAY 12
DAY 13	DAY 14	DAY 15

DAY 16	DAY 17	DAY 18
DAY 19	DAY 20	DAY 21
DAY 22	DAY 23	DAY 24
DAY 25	DAY 26	DAY 27
DAY 28	DAY 29	DAY 30

30-day challenge

DAY 1	DAY 2	DAY 3
DAY 4	DAY 5	DAY 6
DAY 7	DAY 8	DAY 9
DAY 10	DAY 11	DAY 12
DAY 13	DAY 14	DAY 15

DAY 16	DAY 17	DAY 18
DAY 19	DAY 20	DAY 21
DAY 22	DAY 23	DAY 24
DAY 25	DAY 26	DAY 27
DAY 28	DAY 29	DAY 30

30-day challenge

DAY 1	DAY 2	DAY 3
DAY 4	DAY 5	DAY 6
DAY 7	DAY 8	DAY 9
DAY 10	DAY 11	DAY 12
DAY 13	DAY 14	DAY 15

DAY 16	DAY 17	DAY 18
DAY 19	DAY 20	DAY 21
DAY 22	DAY 23	DAY 24
DAY 25	DAY 26	DAY 27
DAY 28	DAY 29	DAY 30

The old me

The new me

notes

Thank you for choosing Soulpress journals.

The Body Joy journal was designed with love especially for you by Soulpress. We hope you'll enjoy it as much as we enjoyed creating it.

If you have any issues with your journal, such as printing errors or faulty binding, please do not hesitate to contact us at **hello@soulpress.co** - we'll make sure you get a replacement copy right away.

For suggestions on how to improve this journal, please get in touch at the same address mentioned above. We'll be happy to take your proposal under consideration and apply it to the next published edition.

If you're happy with your purchase, please share your experience. Your support is greatly appreciated!

Thank you,
Soulpress

Printed in Great Britain
by Amazon